NUCLEAR MEDICINE BOARD REVIEW

Questions and Answers for Self-Assessment

D0879950

NUCLEAR MEDICINE BOARD REVIEW

Questions and Answers for Self-Assessment

C. Richard Goldfarb, M.D.
Editor, Clinical Science
Professor of Radiology
Albert Einstein College of Medicine
Chief, Division of Nuclear Medicine
Beth Israel Medical Center
New York, New York

Jeffrey A. Cooper, M.D.
Contributing Editor
Professor of Radiology and Pediatrics
Director of Nuclear Medicine
Albany Medical Center
Albany, New York

Steven R. Parmett, M.D.
Editor, Clinical Science
Assistant Professor of Clinical Radiology
Columbia University College of Physicians and Surgeons
St. Luke's-Roosevelt Hospital Center
New York, New York

Lionel S. Zuckier, M.D.
Editor, Basic Science
Associate Professor
Nuclear Medicine and Radiology
Albert Einstein College of Medicine
Bronx, New York

1998
Thieme
New York * Stuttgart

Thieme New York
333 Seventh Avenue
New York, New York 10001

Nuclear Medicine Board Review: Questions and Answers for Self-Assessment
C. Richard Goldfarb, M.D., Jeffrey A. Cooper, M.D., Steven R. Parmett, M.D.,
and Lionel S. Zuckier, M.D.

Library of Congress Cataloging-in-Publication Data

Nuclear medicine board review : questions and answers for self
  -assessment / C. Richard Goldfarb, editor, clinical science . . . [et
  al.].
      p.   cm.
   Includes bibliographical references.
   ISBN 0-86577-703-9 — ISBN 3-13-107871-5
   1. Nuclear medicine—Examinations, questions, etc.
  2. Radioisotope scanning—Examinations, questions, etc.
  I. Goldfarb, C. Richard.
   [DNLM: 1. Nuclear Medicine—examination questions.   WN 18.2 N9638
  1998]
  R896.N813   1998
  616.07'575'076—dc21
  DNLM/DLC   97-41323
  for Library of Congress   CIP

Important note: Medical knowledge is ever-changing. As new research and clinical experience broaden our knowledge, changes in treatment and drug therapy may be required. The authors and editors of the material herein have consulted sources believed to be reliable in their efforts to provide information that is complete and in accord with the standards accepted at the time of publication. However, in view of the possibility of human error by the authors, editors, or publisher of the work herein, or changes in medical knowledge, neither the authors, editors, publisher, nor any other party who has been involved in the preparation of this work, warrants that the information contained herein is in every aspect accurate or complete. Readers are encouraged to confirm the information contained herein with other sources. For example, readers are advised to check the product information sheet included in the package of each drug they plan to administer to be certain that the information contained in this publication is accurate and that changes have not been made in the recommended dose or in the contraindications for administration. This recommendation is of particular importance in connection with new or infrequently used drugs.

Some of the product names, patents, and registered designs referred to in this book are in fact registered trademarks or proprietary names even though specific reference to this fact is not always made in the text. Therefore, the appearance of a name without designation is proprietary is not to be construed as a representation by the publisher that it is in the public domain.

Printed in the United States of America

5 4 3
TNY ISBN 0-86577-703-9
GTV ISBN 3-13-107871-5

"To my residents."

Jeffrey A. Cooper

"To Savta and Saba with appreciation for invaluable assistance in fulfilling my editorial responsibilities and for their role in providing me with Ema, Adina, Akiva, Aviva, Aliza, and Atara."

C. Richard Goldfarb

"To Ofra with love and gratitude."

Steven R. Parmett

"Dedicated to my scintillating wife Lydia and energetic children Shlomo, Shira, Tzvi, and Shifra."

Lionel S. Zuckier

Table of Contents

List of Contributors

Steven Braha, M.D.
Brookdale Medical Center
Brooklyn, New York

Jeffrey A. Cooper, M.D.
Albany Medical Center
Albany, New York

Howard Finestone, M.D.
Beth Israel Medical Center
New York, New York

Leonard M. Freeman, M.D.
Montefiore Medical Center
Bronx, New York

Rosemary T. Gallagher, M.A.
Beth Israel Medical Center
New York, New York

C. *Richard Goldfarb, M.D.*
Albert Einstein College of Medicine
Chief, Division of Nuclear Medicine
Beth Israel Medical Center
New York, New York

Gopal Korupolu, M.D.
Spring Hill Medical Center and Doctor's
    Clinic, PA
Spring Hill, Florida

Michael Middleton, M.D.
Scott and White Clinic
Temple, Texas

Justin K. Moran, Ph.D.
Albert Einstein College of Medicine
Bronx, New York

Sumathi Murthy-Wable, M.D.
Medical College of Pennsylvania
    Hospital
Philadelphia, Pennsylvania

Fukiat Ongseng, M.D.
Beth Israel Medical Center
New York, New York

David E. Panzer, M.D.
Mayo Clinic
Jacksonville, Florida

Steven R. Parmett, M.D.
Columbia University College of
    Physicians and Surgeons
St. Luke's-Roosevelt Hospital Center
New York, New York

Serafin Tiu, M.D.
New York University School of Medicine
New York, New York

Michael D. Winn, M.D.
North Shore University Hospital
Forest Hills, New York

Lionel S. Zuckier, M.D.
Albert Einstein College of Medicine
Bronx, New York

Preface

This book evolved out of a perceived need to provide straightforward, accurate review material in nuclear medicine, which could be used for board examinations or general review. We adopted a question and rapid answer format, which was felt to be the most direct and painless method of imparting information. Though not intended to replace textbooks which teach image interpretation, the current work does cover and review much of the basic fund of information which underlies the practice of nuclear medicine, and which is useful for examination. We have also endeavored to include sufficient basic science and quality control material to give the reader a grounding in these important areas as well.

While the quiz format was chosen to accommodate those preparing for board examinations, the vast amount of factual material can serve the needs of course designers, lecturers and residents on nuclear medicine rotation. Our colleagues who sampled the material in pre-published format found it user friendly and suggested its suitability for practicing nuclear physicians who wish to test, update and reinforce their foundation of knowledge.

At some risk of violating the tradition of staid and sober dissemination of sacred scientific information, we adopted some novel approaches to conveying nuclear knowledge. First, there is "instant gratification" of solutions provided within centimeters of problems. Second, two of us (CRG and JAC) provided the intellectual interlude and refreshment of neologisms dispersed among the 1500 or so questions.

We wish you the best of success in using this book, whatever your noble motivation. We'd be pleased to hear from you in regard to its style or content.

C. Richard Goldfarb, M.D.

Jeffrey A. Cooper, M.D.

Steven R. Parmett, M.D.

Lionel S. Zuckier, M.D.

Acknowledgments

We wish to express our gratitude to Mr. Jeffrey Leung for his advice regarding the design of this book. Mr. Daniel Jonas was an invaluable editorial aide while Drs. Konstantin Nikiforov and Mark Guelfguat deserve recognition for their critique of the final manuscript.

Section I
Basic Science

1 Radionuclides and Radiopharmaceuticals

Q: Nuclei with the same atomic number (i.e., protons), but different and numbers of neutrons (i.e., ^{15}O, ^{16}O, ^{17}O) are called _____ .

A: isotopes

Q: Two nuclides with the same atomic mass are called _____ .

A: isobars

Q: Two nuclides with the same number of neutrons are called _____ .

A: isotones

Q: What is a *radionuclide*?

A: a nuclide that emits particulate or photon energy to achieve a more stable energy state

Q: Another name for a helium ion containing two protons and two neutrons is _____ .

A: alpha (α) particle

Q: Why are alpha (α) particles useless for imaging?

A: they cannot exit the body to be detected

Q: What is a beta (β) particle?

A: an electron

Q: What ratio of protons to neutrons favors beta decay?

A: low proton-to-neutron ratio, as compared to stable nuclei

Q: What two particles are emitted from the nucleus with beta decay?

A: a beta (β) particle and an antineutrino

Q: What is the relationship between the mean energy and the maximum energy of a β spectrum?

A: mean energy is approximately one-third the maximum energy

Q: Why are β particles useless for imaging?

A: they cannot exit the body to be detected

Q: What ratio of protons to neutrons favors positron decay?

A: high proton-to-neutron ratio

Q: What particles are released from the nucleus during positron decay?

A: a positron (anti-electron) and a neutrino

Q: What is the minimum nuclear energy required for positron decay?

A: 1.02 meV

Q: What is the fate of a positron?

A: to travel a short distance, combine with an electron, and be annihilated

Q: When a positron is annihilated by interaction with an electron, the result is the production of _____ .

A: two 511 keV photons

Q: What ratio of protons to neutrons favors electron capture decay?

A: high proton-to-neutron ratio

Q: What particle is released from the nucleus during electron capture decay?

A: neutrino

Q: What is released from the nucleus during isomeric transition?

A: gamma rays

Q: The fundamental difference between X rays and gamma rays is that _____ .

A: X rays are produced from energy released due to changes in the orbital electrons of an atom, while gamma rays are produced from energy shifts in the nucleus

Q: When energy from a nuclear transition results in emission of an orbital electron rather than a gamma ray, this process is called _____ .

A: internal conversion

Q: Internal conversion electrons increase patient radiation dose because _____ .

A: energy from the electron is absorbed within the patient's body

Q: When energy from an orbital transition results in emission of an orbital electron rather than an X ray, the particle is called an _____ .

A: Auger electron

Q: What does *metastable* mean?

A: when an isomeric state is long-lived, i.e., longer than 10^{-12} sec

Q: After an electron is ejected from an inner shell, what occurs?

A: electrons in the outer shells collapse to fill the inner shell and give off energy as characteristic X rays

Q: What are the two methods used to create radioactive material that does not occur naturally?

A: bombarding a target material with ions or with neutrons

Q: A _____ is used to bombard elements with neutrons.

A: nuclear reactor

Q: A _____ is used to bombard elements with protons.

A: accelerator (linear or cyclotron)

Q: Examples of four common cyclotron-produced radionuclides in nuclear medicine are _____ .

A: ^{111}In, ^{123}I, ^{67}Ga, and ^{201}Tl

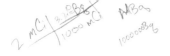

$$2\ mCi \times \frac{3.7\ MBq}{1000\ mCi}$$ MBq

$$\frac{10000083q}$$

Q: What is a *carrier-free* radioisotope?

A: one that does not contain any nonradioactive isotope

Q: What does *activity* mean?

A: the rate of disintegration of a radionuclide

Q: The unit of radioactivity equal to 3.7×10^{10} disintegrations per sec (dps) is called a _____ .

A: curie (Ci)

Q: What is a *becquerel* (Bq)?

A: a unit of radioactivity in the (SI) system equal to 1 dps

Q: A 2 mCi dose of radiopharmaceutical is equivalent to _____ MBq.

A: 74

Q: What does *specific activity* mean?

A: the ratio of activity per unit mass (i.e., mCi/mg, mCi/mole)

Q: The time it takes a radionuclide to decay to one-half its original activity is called the _____ half-life.

A: physical

Q: What is the relationship between physical half-life and the decay constant?

A: their product equals 0.693

Q: The time required for a substance in the body to be reduced in half by biologic excretion or metabolism is called the _____ .

A: biologic half-life

Q: Which type of half-life refers to the overall loss of radioactivity from the body due to physical and biological decay?

A: effective half-life

Q: What is the relationship between effective-half, physical half-life, and biologic half-life?

A: $$\frac{1}{\text{physical half-life}} + \frac{1}{\text{biological half-life}} = \frac{1}{\text{effective half-life}}$$

Q: A radiopharmaceutical with a 6-hour physical half-life and a 3-hour biologic half-life has an effective half-life of _____ .

A: 2 hr

Q: In a parent–daughter generator system, when the half-life of the parent is longer than that of the daughter but not infinite, we have what is called _____ equilibrium.

A: transient

Q: A common example of transient equilibrium is a _____ generator.

A: ^{99}Mo / ^{99m}TcO$_4^-$

Q: When the daughter radionuclide has a half-life longer than that of the parent, we have _____ equilibrium.

A: no

Q: When the parent half-life is very much longer than that of the daughter, we have _____ equilibrium.

A: secular

Q: What are the components of $^{99}Mo/^{99m}Tc$ generator systems?

A: alumina (Al_2O_3) column loaded with ^{99}Mo, an eluting solvent, and an evacuated collecting vial

Q: The source of ^{99}Mo, used for $^{99}Mo/^{99m}Tc$ generators, is from _____ of uranium 235.

A: fission

Q: What is the half-life of ^{99}Mo?

A: 2.8 days (66 hours)

Q: How is a $^{99}Mo/^{99m}Tc$ generator system eluted?

A: ^{99m}Tc is removed by passing saline through the column

Q: Maximum build-up of ^{99m}Tc, in a $^{99}Mo/^{99m}Tc$ generator system, occurs after _____ hours.

A: 23 hr

Q: What does _breakthrough_ mean when applied to a radionuclide generator system?

A: when some parent nuclide (i.e., ^{99}Mo) elutes off the column along with the daughter nuclei (i.e., ^{99m}Tc)

Q: What are the major emissions of ^{99m}Tc?

A: 140 keV photons

Q: By what method does ^{99m}Tc decay?

A: isomeric transition

Q: What is the half-life of ^{99m}Tc?

A: 6 hr

Q: What are the possible valence states of ^{99m}Tc?

A: eight oxidation states from 1− to 7+

Q: What is the valence state and chemical form of ^{99m}Tc eluted from a generator?

A: in pertechnetate (TcO_4^{-1}), Tc is in the 7+ oxidation state

Q: $^{99m}TcO_4^{-1}$ must first be _____ to a valence state of +4 prior to incorporation into most chelates.

A: reduced

Q: Reduction of technetium in commercial radiopharmaceutical kits is generally achieved with _____ .

A: stannous ion

Q: _____ is the single radiopharmaceutical where technetium is _not_ reduced from its 7+ oxidation state.

A: ^{99m}Tc-sulfur colloid

Q: Where does intravenously administered ^{99m}Tc-pertechnetate concentrate?

A: stomach, salivary glands, thyroid, small and large bowel, choroid plexus, lactating breasts, and kidneys

Q: For ^{99m}Tc-macroaggregated albumen (MAA), _____ particles typically are administered.

A: 200,000–500,000

Q: What is the half-life of ^{123}I?

A: 13.2 hr

Q: What is the mode of decay of ^{123}I?

A: electron capture

Q: What are the photons emitted by decay of ^{123}I?

A: 159 keV

Q: What is the half-life of ^{131}I?

A: 8.04 days

Q: What is the mode of decay of ^{131}I?

A: β^- emission

Q: What is the predominant photon emitted by decay of ^{131}I?

A: 364 keV

Q: What is the half-life of ^{133}Xe?

A: 5.3 days

Q: What is the predominant photon emitted by decay of ^{133}Xe?

A: 81 keV

Q: What is the energy of the principle β produced by decay of ^{133}Xe?

A: E_{max} of 346 keV, an E_{mean} of 101 keV

Q: What is the half-life of ^{127}Xe?

A: 36.4 days

Q: What are the predominant photons emitted by decay of ^{127}Xe?

A: 172 keV and 203 keV

Q: What does gallium primarily bind to in plasma?

A: transferrin

Q: What biologically important element does gallium most closely mimic?

A: iron (same oxidation state and similar ionic radius)

Q: What is the half-life of ^{67}Ga?

A: 3.24 days

Q: What are the predominant photons emitted by the decay of ^{67}Ga?

A: 93, 185, 300, and 394 keV

Q: How is gallium excreted?

A: through the kidneys and bowel

Q: What is the main excretory pathway for gallium in the first 24 hours?

A: urine (10% of administered dose)

Q: What is the half-life of ^{111}In?

A: 2.83 days

Q: What are the predominant photons emitted by the decay of ^{111}In?

A: 171 keV and 245 keV

Q: What are three important uses of ^{111}In?

A: labeling of leukocytes, antibodies, and peptides

Q: In addition to ^{111}In, monoclonal antibodies, for clinical use, have been labeled with _____ .

A: ^{99m}Tc

Q: The first several FDA-approved antibodies are based on monoclonal antibodies derived from what species?

A: mouse

Q: A repeat administration of a murine-derived antibody may result in _____ .

A: accelerated clearance due to presence of human anti-mouse antibodies (HAMA)

Q: Antibodies bind to _____ on tumors.

A: antigens or epitopes

Q: ^{111}In-labeled Pentreotide (Octreoscan) is an example of a class of imaging agents called _____ .

A: peptides

Q: Pentreotide binds to a _____ on the surface of a tumor.

A: somatostatin receptor

Q: Octreotide, the peptide that is labeled in Octreoscan, is _____ amino acids in length.

A: 8

Q: What is the half-life of ^{201}Tl?

A: 3.08 days

Q: What are the predominant photons emitted by the decay of ^{201}Tl?

A: mercury X rays of 69–71 keV and 80 keV

Q: What is the mechanism of ^{201}Tl decay?

A: electron capture

Q: What is the usual chemical form of ^{201}Tl?

A: thallous chloride (TlCl)

Q: What biologically important ion does ^{201}Tl most closely mimic?

A: potassium (same charge and similar ionic radius)

Q: What is the principle utility of positron-emitting radionuclides?

A: positron-emitting radionuclides are used for positron emission tomography (PET), where coincident gamma rays are detected

Q: The main technical difficulty with positron emission tomography (PET) radionuclides is that they tend to have a very _____ half-life.

A: short

Q: Positron-emitting radionuclides, as used in PET scanning, tend to be produced by generator systems or by an on-site _____ .

A: cyclotron

Q: ^{18}F-flouro-deoxyglucose (FDG) is an analog of _____ , which is taken up by cells and phosphorylated but cannot be further processed.

A: glucose

Q: The property of ^{18}F-FDG that makes it useful for imaging tumors is that _____ .

A: tumors derive energy from metabolism of glucose more so than other tissues

Q: ^{82}Rb, used for PET myocardial perfusion studies, is obtained from a _____ generator.

A: ^{82}Sr

Q: The mechanism of localization in _____ is achieved by capillary blockage.

A: perfusion lung scanning

Q: Bone scintigraphic agents localize by the process of _____ .

A: adsorption onto hydroxyapatite

Q: A common positron-emitting radiopharmaceutical that localizes by active transport is _____ .

A: ^{18}F-FDG

Q: A radiopharmaceutical that localizes by phagocytosis is _____ .

A: ^{99m}Tc-sulfur colloid

Q: Antibody-imaging agents localize by _____ .

A: antigen-antibody binding

Q: Somatostatin analogues localize by _____ .

A: receptor binding

Q: ^{89}Sr chloride (metastron) is a therapeutic radiopharmaceutical used to treat _____ .

A: pain of bony metastases

Q: ^{89}Sr, a β^- emitter, decays with a physical half-life of _____ days.

A: 50.5

Q: The photons produced in an annihilation are oriented at a _____ angle to each other.

A: 180°

Q: ^{11}C, ^{13}N, ^{15}O, and ^{18}F are all produced by _____ .

A: cyclotron

Q: In PET imaging, attenuation correction can be made by placing a source in the scanner and generating a _____ scan.

A: transmission

Q: The _____ technique at image reconstruction permits the use of the relative timing of scintillation in two detectors recording a coincidence to approximate the exact site of a positron annihilation.

A: time of flight

Q: Annihilation usually occurs on the order of several _____ from the site of emission of the positron.

A: millimeters

Q: The half-life of ^{18}F is _____ .

A: 110 min

2 Instrumentation

Q: What is a gamma camera crystal made of?

A: sodium iodide activated with thallium

Q: What is the purpose of the crystal in a gamma camera?

A: to absorb gamma rays and convert them into visible light photons

Q: What is the mechanism by which gamma rays interact with a gamma camera crystal?

A: photoelectric effect or compton scattering

Q: What is the relationship between the energy of an absorbed gamma ray and the amount of light produced by a gamma camera crystal?

A: the amount of light produced is directly proportional to the amount of energy lost by the absorbed gamma ray

Q: What is the purpose of the photomultiplier tube (PMT) array?

A: to detect the light photons produced in the crystal and produce a proportional pulse

Q: How does increasing crystal thickness influence camera sensitivity and resolution?

A: thick crystals (i.e., 1/2 inch) have higher sensitivity but lower resolution

Q: What is the output of a single PMT?

A: a pulse (very small signal) that represents amplification of the light detected

Q: The PMTs are _____ to the crystal by optical grease or a light pipe

A: optically coupled

Q: What is the output of the PMT array decoder circuit?

A: spatial coordinates $(x+, x-, y+, y-)$ of the scintillation event

Q: Increasing the number of PMTs _____ resolution.

A: improves

Q: How many PMTs are in a modern gamma camera?

A: 75 or 91 per head

Q: The electronic component in a gamma camera that is used to eliminate unwanted photons is called a _____ .

A: pulse height analyzer

Q: Why do scattered photons from within the patient cause major imaging difficulties?

A: scattered photons lead to incorrectly positioned radioactive events

Q: What is the *window* in a pulse height analyzer (PHA)?

A: range of acceptable energies around a photopeak

Q: What are the energy limits of a 20% window centered at 140 keV?

A: 126keV–154keV

Q: Why do some gamma camera have multiple PHAs?

A: to simultaneously acquire several peaks (i.e., ^{67}Ga)

Q: What are the advantages of a digital camera?

A: better energy and spatial resolution, less dead time

Q: Digital gamma cameras use a _____ to apply prestored energy and position corrections to each scintillation event.

A: computer

Q: What is a gamma camera collimator made of?

A: lead or tungsten

Q: What is the purpose of a gamma camera collimator?

A: to project an image of the source distribution directly onto the crystal

Q: What does *collimator sensitivity* mean?

A: ratio of gamma rays that pass through the collimator to those incident upon it

Q: When is it appropriate to use a pinhole collimator?

A: when imaging small organs that lie close to the body surface (e.g., thyroid)

Q: What are the principle disadvantages of a pinhole collimator?

A: image distortion and poor sensitivity

Q: As a pinhole collimator is brought closer to an object being imaged, the apparent size of the object _____ .

A: increases

Q: As a pinhole collimator is brought closer to an object being imaged, resolution _____ .

A: improves

Q: As a pinhole collimator is brought closer to an object being imaged, count-rate _____ .

A: increases

Q: What is the most common type of collimator hole alignment in nuclear medicine?

A: parallel hole

Q: As a parallel-hole collimator is brought closer to an object being imaged, resolution _____ .

A: improves

Q: As a parallel-hole collimator is brought closer to an object being imaged, the apparent size of the object _____ .

A: stays the same

Q: As a parallel-hole collimator is brought closer to an object being imaged, count-rate _____ .

A: remains the same

Q: Walls within the collimator that separate adjacent holes are called _____ .

A: collimator septa

Q: What is the purpose of collimator septa?

A: to block gamma rays that are travelling obliquely towards the crystal

Q: What does *septal penetration* mean?

A: gamma rays passing obliquely through collimator septa leading to mispositioned events

Q: Presence of a *starburst* type appearance when imaging a hot object with a parallel hole collimator is due to _____ .

A: septal penetration

Q: What defines the energy range of a collimator?

A: composition, thickness, and length of the septa

Q: How does increasing septal length affect collimator resolution and sensitivity?

A: improves resolution and lowers sensitivity

Q: How does increasing septal thickness affect collimator energy?

A: permits use of higher energy gamma emitters

Q: What is the shape of holes currently used in parallel-hole collimators and why?

A: hexagonal holes can be more closely packed, thereby covering a greater area of the detector face

Q: How should a parallel-hole collimator be positioned relative to the patient for best resolution?

A: as close as possible

Q: A measure of the ability of the camera to separate events of different energies is called _____ .

A: energy resolution

Q: A measure of the ability of an imaging system to distinguish two adjacent point sources as distinct is called _____ .

A: spatial resolution

Q: What does *intrinsic resolution* mean?

A: resolution due to all components of the gamma camera system except the collimator

Q: What is the difference between intrinsic and overall (or *extrinsic*) resolution?

A: extrinsic resolution includes the effect of the collimator

Q: Typical intrinsic resolution for a modern gamma camera is _____ .

A: 3–8 mm

Q: How does intrinsic resolution vary with photon energy?

A: intrinsic resolution decreases as energy drops below an optimal energy range

Q: The time it takes electronics of the system to reset after an event is called _____ .

A: dead time

Q: In what type of studies is dead time most important?

A: high count rate studies (e.g., cardiac first pass)

Q: The typical dead time for a modern gamma camera is _____ .

A: 5–10 μsec

Q: The basic principle of single photon emission computed tomography (SPECT) is _____ .

A: by imaging in multiple planes around a subject, the original count distribution can be reconstructed using the mathematical algorithm of filtered back-projection

Q: How is an conventional planar gamma camera modified to accomplish SPECT?

A: the camera head is made to rotate around the patient and is interfaced to a computer that reconstructs the data in 3D

Q: The acquisition method by which the camera rotates by several degrees, acquires in a stationary position, and repeats is called _____ .

A: step and shoot

Q: The purpose of noncircular or elliptical orbits in SPECT imaging is _____ .

A: improve spatial resolution by decreasing patient–collimator distance

Q: The advantage of multiple heads in a SPECT system is an increase in _____ .

A: count-rate sensitivity and decrease in imaging time

Q: The major disadvantage of multiple heads in a SPECT system is difficulty in _____ .

A: alignment and registration of the multiple heads

Q: What factor limits the total acquisition time of a SPECT study?

A: patient movement and fatigue

Q: What is the most common algorithm used for reconstructing tomographic images in a SPECT study?

A: filtered back projection

Q: What is the advantage of filtered back projection over unfiltered back projection?

A: elimination of the starburst artifact—apparent streaks emanating from a point source upon reconstruction

Q: What is an image filter?

A: mathematical technique used to eliminate unwanted components in the projection profiles from appearing in the reconstructed image

Q: What is the filter used specifically in filtered back projection?

A: modified ramp filter, e.g., Hanning, shepp-logan, butterworth

Q: When can filtering be performed in SPECT processing?

A: either prereconstruction (2D) or postreconstruction (3D)

Q: Why do computers use the binary system?

A: digital computers are based on circuits made from semiconductor materials where numbers are stored as series of on and off signals representing ones and zeros

Q: What is the binary number system?

A: a base-two numbering system, composed of 0s and 1s and built upon powers of 2

Q: What is the binary number 10011 in the decimal system?

A: $(1 \times 16) + (0 \times 8) + (0 \times 4) + (1 \times 2) + (1 \times 1) = 19$

Q: What is a computer program?

A: a series of lines of computer code that causes the computer hardware to perform a specific task

Q: The section of the computer memory that contains instructions that can be read but not changed by the user is called _____ .

A: read-only memory (ROM)

Q: The section of the computer memory that provides a temporary storage for program instructions and data is called _____ .

A: random-access memory (RAM)

3 Quality Control

Q: The percentage of radioactivity in a preparation originating from the desired radionuclide is called _____ purity.

A: radionuclidic

Q: The maximum permissible amount of ^{99}Mo per mCi of ^{99m}Tc _____ .

A: 0.15 μCi per mCi ^{99m}Tc, with a maximum of 2.5 μCi total, at time of administration

Q: The radionuclidic purity of ^{99m}Tc _____ during the day because of the longer physical half-life of ^{99}Mo compared to ^{99m}Tc.

A: decreases

Q: An important cause of impurity in ^{123}I preparations is _____ .

A: ^{124}I

Q: A multichannel analyzer may be used to assess radionuclidic purity by evaluation of the _____ of the sample.

A: energy spectrum

Q: The energy of ^{99}Mo photons are _____ .

A: 740 keV and 780 keV

Q: A simple common method used to evaluate for presence of ^{99}Mo in ^{99m}Tc samples is by use of a dose calibrator and _____ .

A: a lead shield (pig) to differentially absorb the low energy photons but allow the energetic ^{99}Mo photons to pass

Q: The percentage of total radioactivity present in a preparation in the desired chemical form is called the _____ purity.

A: radiochemical

Q: Presence of free ^{99m}TcO$_4$$^{-1}$ in a ^{99m}Tc-red blood cell (RBC) preparation is an example of a _____ impurity.

A: radiochemical

Q: In $^{99m}TcO_4^{-1}$ preparations, the three general forms of technetium are free pertechnetate, chelated technetium, and _____ .

A: reduced hydrolyzed technetium

Q: Reduced hydrolyzed technetium has a tendency to be taken up by the _____ .

A: liver

Q: The form of technetium that is concentrated by the thyroid and gastric mucosa is _____ .

A: $^{99m}TcO_4^{-1}$

Q: If it is suspected that gastric activity on a bleeding scan is a result of free pertechnetate, one should image the _____ to confirm.

A: thyroid

Q: The most common means of evaluating radiochemical purity is by use of _____ .

A: instant thin layer chromatography

Q: As a general rule of thumb for radiopharmaceuticals made with $^{99m}TcO_4^{-1}$, radiochemical purity should be _____ .

A: not less than 90%

Q: _____ purity refers to presence of nonradioactive compounds in a preparation that may interfere with normal behavior or safety of the radiopharmaceutical.

A: chemical

Q: A common source of chemical impurity, originating from the $^{99}Mo/^{99m}TcO_4^{-1}$ generator, is _____ .

A: aluminum from the alumina column

Q: Presence of excess amounts of aluminum in a ^{99m}Tc-sulfur colloid preparation leads to excess uptake in the _____ .

A: lungs

Q: Presence of excess amounts of aluminum in a ^{99m}Tc-methylene diphosphonate (MDP) preparation leads to excess uptake in the _____ .

A: liver

Q: Presence of aluminum in a generator eluate can be tested by _____ .

A: indicator paper (aurintricarboxylic acid)

Q: Permissible quantities of aluminum in a fission ^{99}Mo generator eluate are _____ .

A: <10 μg/ml eluate

Q: Presence of excess amounts of stannous ion in a ^{99m}Tc-MDP preparation leads to excess uptake in the _____ .

A: liver

Q: ^{32}P-sodium phosphate, used for treatment of polycythemia vera by intravenous (IV) injection, appears _____ .

A: clear and colorless

Q: ^{32}P-chromic phosphate, used in the treatment of malignant ascites by intra-peritoneal (IP) injection, appears _____ .

A: greenish-blue and turbid

Q: Macroaggregated albumin should be of what particle size?

A: 90% between 10 and 90 μm diameter

Q: Sulfur colloid should be of what particle size?

A: 0.1 to 1 μm

Q: Fever-producing toxins, which often originate in gram-negative bacteria and may contaminate radiopharmaceuticals, are called _____ .

A: pyrogens

Q: The rapid method of testing for pyrogens is by the _____ .

A: limulus amebocyte lysate assay, using the blood of the horseshoe crab

Q: The formal method of testing for pyrogens is by _____ .

A: injection of the sample into rabbits and monitoring their temperature

Q: For radiopharmaceuticals administered into the cerebrospinal fluid (CSF), endotoxin is _____ toxic than in systemically administered preparations.

A: much more

Q: Absence of viable microbes within a radiopharmaceutical is called _____ .

A: sterility

Q: The phenomenon of increased counts at the periphery of the scintillation crystal, due to internal reflection of light at the edges, is called _____ .

A: edge packing

Q: Uniformity flood images of each gamma camera should be performed on a _____ basis.

A: daily

Q: The difference between a gamma camera intrinsic flood and extrinsic flood is that the intrinsic flood is _____ .

A: performed without the collimator

Q: The advantage for using a cobalt source rather than liquid-filled phantom for performing floods is _____ .

A: more constant thickness and no air bubbles

Q: When performing intrinsic floods using a point source, the point source should be located at least _____ away from the crystal to ensure a homogenous distribution of radiation across the crystal face.

A: 5 crystal diameters

Q: When the aluminum cover around a scintillation crystal is breached, the flood images can appear spotty ("measles") because of _____ of the crystal.

A: hygroscopic degeneration

Q: The effect of a nonfunctioning PMT on a flood field is _____ .

A: presence of a discrete cold region

Q: The term for tuning an energy window to the spectrum of a given isotope is _____ .

A: peaking

Q: The width of the measured spectrum for a particular gamma peak is a measure of the _____ of the gamma camera.

A: energy resolution

Q: Peaking of the camera should be performed on a _____ basis.

A: daily

Q: The ability of a gamma camera to resolve objects close together is called the _____ .

A: spatial resolution

Q: Spatial resolution should be tested on a _____ basis.

A: weekly

Q: Spatial resolution is generally tested by imaging _____ .

A: bar phantoms

Q: The ability of the gamma camera to portray straight lines as straight is called _____ .

A: spatial linearity

Q: As a general rule, spatial linearity should be tested on a _____ basis.

A: weekly

Q: Difficulty in scaling size of images taken at multiple energy peaks (i.e., ^{67}Ga) is due to problems in _____ .

A: z-pulse normalization

Q: When SPECT imaging is performed with a gamma camera, the need for uniformity on the flood images is _____ , compared with planar imaging.

A: greater

Q: Why should quality assurance of a SPECT gamma camera be stricter than a planar gamma camera?

A: a 1% nonuniformity in planar images have been shown to amplify to 20% nonuniformity in the reconstructed SPECT images

Q: A _____ reconstruction artifact occurs with a nonuniform SPECT camera.

A: bulls-eye

Q: How many counts should be obtained for a SPECT gamma camera uniformity flood?

A: 64 ×64 matrix should have 30 million counts, while a 128 ×128 matrix should have 120 million counts

Q: Should a uniformity flood on a SPECT gamma camera be done intrinsically or extrinsically?

A: extrinsically

Q: For SPECT cameras, an additional quality control measure is verifying the _____ .

A: center of rotation

Q: How is center of rotation data used in SPECT gamma cameras?

A: for reconstructing 3D images

Q: How accurate must the center of rotation be?

A: optimally within half a pixel

Q: How can the overall system performance of a SPECT camera be evaluated?

A: acquire images of a SPECT phantom, for example a Jaszczak phantom

Q: The minimal intrinsic resolution, linearity, and uniformity of a SPECT gamma camera should be _____ .

A: intrinsic resolution of 3–4 mm full width half maximum (FWHM), intrinsic linearity of 0.2–0.6 mm, and intrinsic uniformity of 2–3%

Q: Before administration, every radiopharmaceutical must be assayed in a _____ .

A: dose calibrator

Q: A dose calibrator operates on the principle of an _____ chamber.

A: ionization

Q: The linearity of a dose calibrator refers to the _____ .

A: accuracy of measurement over the range of activities counted in the dose calibrator, i.e., 1 mCi to 1000 Ci

Q: As a general rule, linearity of a dose calibrator should be tested on a _____ basis.

A: quarterly

Q: The simplest way to test for linearity of the dose calibrator is _____ .

A: by counting a large dose of ^{99m}Tc over a period of multiple half-lives

Q: A rapid method of testing linearity is by _____ .

A: counting a large sample of ^{99m}Tc with and without attenuation by calibrated lead sleeves

Q: Geometry of a dose calibrator refers to the relationship between _____ .

A: measured activity and the position and shape of the source within the counting chamber

Q: Geometry of a dose calibrator should be tested _____ .

A: at installation and after major repair work

Q: Constancy (or precision) of measurement in a dose calibrator refers to the _____ .

A: reproducibility of measurement over long periods of time

Q: Dose calibrator constancy is evaluated by _____ .

A: comparing interval measurements of a known standard source, e.g., ^{137}Cs, both at its own settings as well as settings of other frequently used isotopes

Q: Constancy should be tested on a _____ basis.

A: daily

Q: According to (NRC) regulations, constancy should be at least

_____ .

A: within 90%

Q: _____ refers to agreement with calibrated values when measuring standards traceable to the National Bureau of Standards.

A: accuracy

Q: Accuracy must be performed on a _____ basis.

A: daily

Q: Accuracy is performed by

_____ .

A: comparing measurements with expected values for at least two different radionuclide standards, such as ^{137}Cs and ^{57}Co, which are traceable to the National Bureau of Standards

Q: According to NRC regulations, accuracy of at least _____ % is required.

A: 90

Q: Comparing the dose calibrator with the sodium-iodide well counter, only the _____ can differentiate the energies of different isotopes.

A: well counter

Q: When simultaneously counting two isotopes in a well counter, such as ^{57}Co and ^{58}Co, *spilldown* refers to _____ .

A: the contribution of counts from the higher energy isotope into the lower energy window

Q: When performing two separate radionuclide imaging procedures on the same patient on the same day, the study using the higher energy isotope should generally be performed _____ .

A: second

Q: Because of statistical variation in radioactive emissions, the standard deviation of a count of 900 counts is

_____ .

A: 30, the square root of n

Q: Radiation-absorbed dose refers to
_____ .

A: the amount of energy deposited per gram of absorbing tissue

Q: Units of radiation dose are the
_____ .

A: rad and the gray

Q: Dose equivalent, measured by the _____ , refers to the radiation-absorbed dose multiplied by a quality factor that compensates for the particular type of radiation involved.

A: rem

Q: Units of exposure, which refer to the level of ionization in air, are the
_____ .

A: roentgen

Q: What is the purpose of a dose calibrator?

A: to measure or verify the activity of all patient doses, generator eluates, or any other large amount (mCi) of radioactive materials by conversion of the ionization current to a display of the radionuclide activity (Bq, Ci)

Q: Why can't a well counter substitute for a dose calibrator?

A: because of the high detection efficiency of a well counter, dead time problems exist for levels of activity greater than $1 \, \mu\text{Ci}$

Q: Why must a dose calibrator be recalibrated for each radionuclide to be measured?

A: a dose calibrator has no energy discriminator components—it functions by measurement of the ionization current. This current is then converted to activity by use of a predetermined calibration factor specific to each isotope

Q: ALARA refers to _____ .

A: the philosophy of limiting occupational exposure from radionuclides to levels *as low as reasonably achievable*

Q: Occupational dose limits for a radiation worker are _____ rem/year.

A: 5

Q: Occupational dose limits for the embryo/fetus of a pregnant radiation worker are _____ rem/year.

A: 0.5

Q: Dose limits for nonradiation workers have been lowered to _____ rem/year.

A: 0.1

Section II
Clinical Science

4 Bone

Q: What are the two main advantages of bone scintigraphy?

A: high sensitivity to early disease and ease of surveying the entire skeleton

Q: What is the main disadvantage of bone scintigraphy?

A: the findings are often nonspecific

Q: What two factors give skeletal scintigraphy its specificity?

A: the clinical context and the total body pattern

Q: What class of radiopharmaceutical compounds are most commonly used for skeletal scintigraphy?

A: ^{99m}Tc-diphosphonates

Q: Why are ^{99m}Tc-diphosphonates superior to ^{99m}Tc-pryophoshates for skeletal scintigraphy?

A: ^{99m}Tc-diphosphonates have faster clearance

Q: How are ^{99m}Tc-diphosphonates prepared?

A: sodium pertechnetate ($NaTcO^4$) from ^{99}Mo- generator is added to vial with diphosphonate and stannous ion, Sn(II). The stannous ion reduces Tc and the reduced Tc chelates to diphosphonate

Q: How does the introduction of oxygen into a vial of ^{99m}Tc-diphosphonate affect the bone scan image?

A: the formation of colloidal Tc causes liver and spleen uptake. The formation of free Tc causes stomach and thyroid uptake.

Q: What is the maximum length of time that should be allowed between preparation and use of ^{99m}Tc-diphosphonates?

A: 2–3 hrs

Q: What percent of a ^{99m}Tc-diphosphonate dose localizes in bone?

A: 50%

Q: How is ^{99m}Tc-diphosphonate that does not localize in bone cleared from the body?

A: glomerular filtration

Q: What percent of the dose is in the blood at 2–3 hrs after injection?

A: 3–5%

Q: What is the mechanism of ^{99m}Tc-diphosphonate localization in bone?

A: adsorption to mineral phase of bone

Q: Why does ^{99m}Tc-diphosphonate have an affinity for newly formed bone?

A: it has higher adsorption to amorphous $CaPO_4$ than to mature hydroxyapatite

Q: What two factors affect the degree of ^{99m}Tc-diphosphonate in bone?

A: bone formation and blood flow

Q: What is the critical organ for radiation dose in skeletal scintigraphy?

A: the bladder

Q: How can a patient decrease the radiation dose from a bone scan?

A: void frequently

Q: How should a patient be prepared for a bone scan?

A: the patient should be well hydrated, void immediately before study, remove metal objects (jewelry, coins, keys) before imaging, and void frequently after the procedure

Q: What is the usual adult dosage and route of administration of ^{99m}Tc-diphosphonates?

A: 20 mCi IV

Q: What special type of imaging should be performed for suspected osteomyelitis versus cellulitis with a bone scan?

A: dynamic blood flow and immediate images

Q: When is delayed imaging performed for bone scanning?

A: at 2–4 hrs after tracer injection

Q: How many counts are typically obtained for spot bone scan images?

A: 600K counts of anterior chest for spot views and all other views for the same time

Q: What type of collimators are used for bone scanning?

A: all-purpose collimator used for routine imaging; high-resolution, pinhole, or converging for more detail

Q: How do child/adolescent bone scans differ from adult bone scans?

A: epiphyseal uptake is present

Q: How do neonatal bone scans differ from child/adolescent bone scans?

A: there is diffusely decreased uptake

Q: How can you tell if the kidneys have increased uptake on a bone scan?

A: the uptake will be more than the lumbar spine uptake

Q: What are four normal variants seen in the skull?

A: uneven or variable uptake, hyperostosis frontalis interna, sphenoid uptake, and uptake between orbits

Q: What is the usual cause of normal anterior neck uptake?

A: laryngotracheal cartilage calcification

Q: Why can joints show mild diffuse asymmetry?

A: handedness

Q: What joints can normally show increased uptake?

A: sternomanubrial joint, sternal ossification centers, sacroiliac joints

Q: Why are axial skeletal metastases most common with epithelial tumors?

A: these tumors typically spread to red marrow first

Q: What is the mechanism of increased bone scan uptake with a bone metastasis?

A: growth of tumor causes surrounding bony remodeling

Q: How much change in bone density is required to see a skeletal metastasis on plain radiography?

A: 30–50%

Q: When can metastatic disease not cause the bone scan to be abnormal?

A: when there is an indolent tumor or a markedly lytic lesion

Q: What is the sensitivity of bone scanning for skeletal metastases?

A: >95%

Q: What is the disadvantage of using magnetic resonance imaging (MRI) to detect bone metastases?

A: it is not feasible to scan entire skeleton, and it is difficult to distinguish heterogeneity in marrow fat or benign defects from metastasis

Q: What is the typical scintigraphic pattern of metastatic disease?

A: multiple focal lesions distributed randomly in the axial skeleton

Q: Why can metastatic disease show a ring lesion on skeletal scintigraphy?

A: uptake is in the reactive bone surrounding a large tumor; the tumor itself does not take up tracer

Q: How can the bone scan findings of osteomalacia and Cushing's syndrome be distinguished from metastatic disease?

A: there is a predominance of rib lesions in osteomalacia and Cushing's syndrome

Q: How can osteoarthritis be distinguished from skeletal metastases on a bone scan?

A: osteoarthritis causes uptake limited to joints commonly involving both sides of a joint

Q: How can trauma to the ribs be distinguished from skeletal metastases on a bone scan?

A: the lesions are aligned

Q: How can Paget's disease be distinguished from skeletal metastases on a bone scan?

A: In Paget's disease, uptake is characteristically intense, and expansile and tracks along the length of a bone or hemipelvis

Q: What are four clues to the diagnosis of a superscan?

A: good bone-to-soft tissue uptake, absent or faint kidney uptake, increased axial-to-appendicular uptake ratio, and findings on plain radiographs

Q: What is a "flare phenomenon"?

A: increased uptake following chemotherapy due to healing of bone after regression of metastases

Q: How long does it usually take for the flare phenomena to normalize?

A: 6 months

Q: Which five tumors commonly metastasize to bone?

A: prostate, breast, lung, kidney, and thyroid

Q: What is the mechanism of cold lesions on a bone scan?

A: loss of blood flow or complete destruction of bone

Q: What two types of tumors tend to cause no bony reaction on a bone scan?

A: multiple myeloma and round cell tumors

Q: What is the usual cause of positive lesions on a bone scan in a patient with multiple myeloma?

A: pathologic fractures

Q: What is the sensitivity of an increased alkaline phosphatase for skeletal metastases from prostate cancer?

A: 50%

Q: What is the sensitivity of plain radiographs for skeletal metastases from prostate cancer?

A: 70%

Q: What percentage of Stage I prostate cancer patients have skeletal metastases on bone scan?

A: 5%

Q: What percentage of Stage I breast cancer patients have skeletal metastases on bone scan?

A: 3–5%

Q: How does mastectomy affect the bone scan?

A: asymmetry of rib uptake

Q: What is the significance of sternal bone scan uptake ipsilateral to a primary breast cancer?

A: it indicates local invasion from metastases to inframammary nodes

Q: Which patients with lung cancer who are being considered for curative surgical resection should get a bone scan?

A: all of them

Q: How does the typical distribution of metastatic disease from lung cancer differ from metastatic disease from breast or prostate cancer?

A: appendicular involvement is more common

Q: What nonmetastatic finding is commonly seen on the bone scan of patients with lung cancer?

A: hypertrophic pulmonary osteoarthropathy

Q: What is the typical location of skeletal metastases of neuroblastoma?

A: metaphysis adjacent to the epiphyseal growth plate

Q: What percentage of primary neuroblastomas take up the tracer on bone scanning?

A: 30–50%

Q: What is the usual age group affected by osteoid osteoma?

A: adolescents and young adults

Q: What is the appearance of osteoid osteoma on bone scanning?

A: hot spot at site of pain

Q: What is the typical uptake of most benign tumors of bone?

A: mildly increased uptake

Q: What types of benign bone tumors can have marked uptake?

A: osteoblastomas and osteoid osteomas

Q: When do enchondromas have markedly increased uptake?

A: when they are complicated by fracture

Q: What percentage of fractures visualize on bone scan by 24 hours?

A: 80%

Q: What percentage of fractures in patients under age 65 visualize on bone scan by 72 hours?

A: 95%

Q: When is fracture sensitivity maximal on bone scan in patients over age 65?

A: at more than 7 days

Q: What percent of nondisplaced uncomplicated fractures are normal at 1 year?

A: 60–80%

Q: What percent of nondisplaced uncomplicated fractures are normal at 3 years?

A: 95%

Q: How long does it take for complicated or displaced fractures to return to normal on bone scan?

A: they are positive indefinitely

Q: How does a craniotomy site present on bone scan?

A: ring pattern that persists for months

Q: How does rib retraction during a thoracotomy affect a bone scan?

A: it causes rib uptake from periosteal reaction

Q: What do intercalary bone grafts look like on bone scan?

A: uptake at bone ends that gradually fill in as graft revitalizes

Q: What do pedicle bone grafts look like on bone scan?

A: diffuse immediate uptake

Q: How does radiation therapy affect bone scan uptake at the site of radiation?

A: initially causes mildly increased uptake with persistently decreased uptake within 6 months to 1 year in the geometric pattern of a radiation port

Q: What is the typical appearance of stress fractures?

A: oval or fusiform uptake that is parallel to long axis of bone

Q: What is the typical appearance of shin splints?

A: diffuse uptake along greater than one-third of the bone length of the mid to distal tibia without focal uptake

Q: What is the prognostic difference between stress fractures and shin splints?

A: stress fractures are predictive of further injury without relief of stress, while shin splints are not predictive of further injury

Q: What is the appearance of rhabdomyolysis on bone scan?

A: localization of tracer in damaged skeletal muscle corresponding to the muscle group that was overexercised

Q: When is the maximum bone scan uptake with rhabdomyolysis?

A: after 24–48 hours

Q: How long does it take for rhabdomyolysis to resolve on bone scan?

A: 1 week

Q: What is the appearance of newly infarcted bone on bone scan?

A: a cold lesion

Q: What imaging technique should be used to detect the osteonecrosis of Legg-Calve-Perthes disease on bone scan?

A: pinhole collimation

Q: What is the typical finding of Legg-Calve-Perthes disease on bone scan early in the course of the disease?

A: a lentiform photon deficient area in upper outer femoral head

Q: What is the typical finding of Legg-Calve-Perthes disease on bone scan midphase in the course of the disease?

A: uptake at margin of photon deficient in the upper outer femoral head

Q: What is the typical finding of Legg-Calve-Perthes disease on bone scan late in the course of the disease?

A: increased uptake in the femoral head

Q: What is the typical finding of steroid-induced osteonecrosis on bone scan?

A: increased uptake in the femoral head

Q: What are five findings of sickle cell disease on bone scan?

A: diffusely increased uptake in calvarium, more appendicular uptake than normal, good skeleton-to-background uptake, kidneys larger than normal, and splenic uptake due to prior infarction

Q: What variation of a routine bone scan should be performed in the differentiation of osteomyelitis from cellulitis?

A: three phase scan

Q: How does one acquire the images for the first phase of a three phase bone scan?

A: inject tracer as bolus and obtain dynamic 2 sec images for 60 sec

Q: How does one acquire the images for the second phase of a three phase bone scan?

A: obtain 600K static images of the area immediately after the first phase

Q: What is the third phase of a three phase bone scan?

A: routine delayed images

Q: How do osteomyelitis and cellulitis differ on the first (flow) phase of a three phase bone scan?

A: osteomyelitis shows arterial hyperemia, cellulitis shows venous hyperemia

Q: How do osteomyelitis and cellulitis differ on the third (skeletal) phase of a three phase bone scan?

A: osteomyelitis shows focal skeletal uptake, cellulitis shows mildly diffused nonfocal uptake

Q: What is the typical appearance of a loose hip joint prosthesis on bone scan?

A: increased uptake at greater and lesser trochanter with increased uptake at prosthesis tip

Q: What is the best scintigraphic method to distinguish between prosthesis loosening and infection?

A: white blood cell scan

Q: What two metabolic bone diseases can show stomach and lung uptake on bone scan? Why?

A: primary hyperparathyroidism and renal osteodystrophy; hypercalcemia with calcium deposition in low PH regions.

Q: What is the role of bone scan in patients with osteoporosis?

A: to detect and date insufficient fractures

Q: How is the bone scan useful in the evaluation of myositis ossificans?

A: degree of uptake diminishes with maturity of the site of calcification; mature lesions can be resected surgically

Q: What do you call the otherworldly flash that a photocopying machine makes as it starts to produce a copy?

A: a) *Copyroxysm*
    b) *Flash in the Scan*
    c) *Flashsimilie*
    d) *Eeriedescence*
    e) *Foreflasher*
    f) *Copyulation Explosion*

Q: Which apply to osteoid osteomas?
a. approximately four times more common in males than in females
b. occur predominately between the ages of 10 and 30
c. the most common locations are in the femur and tibia

A: all are correct

Q: In osteoid osteomas, the bone scan will show _____ .

A: "double-density" sign, an area of diffusely increased uptake, with a focal area of more avid uptake

Q: Osteogenic sarcoma commonly shows a photon-deficient pattern when it occurs in _____ bone.

A: pagetic

Q: True/false: With breast carcinoma, flare response is seen in patients who responded to therapy as compared with nonresponders.

A: true

Q: In prostate cancer patients, low levels of PSA correlate with a very low likelihood of bone metastasis, except in those who have had _____ treatment.

A: hormonal

Q: True/false: Bone labeling is not increased significantly after 30 min.

A: true

Q: *Spot view* resolution generally outperforms *whole-body* acquisition resolution by large detectors capable of single-pass acquisitions. Why?

A: the crystal is closer to the patient

Q: Metastatic calcification shows intense labeling of the _____ .

A: lungs and the fundus of the stomach

Q: True/false: In Paget's disease that appears lytic on x-ray, photopenia is common on bone scan.

A: false

Q: True/false: Extremely intense labeling is characteristic of fibrous dysplasia.

A: true

Q: True/false: In acute osteomyelitis, blood flow is increased in the arterial phase.

A: true

Q: Neutrophils are resistant to radiation from ^{111}In labeling, whereas lymphocytes are very sensitive to ^{111}In radiation damage. What is the clinical implication?

A: a lymphocytic response to chronic infection is not excluded by this technique

Q: ^{99m}Tc _____ is superior to other currently used bone agents at localizing necrotic tissue.

A: pyrophosphate

Q: Vertical linear activity in the posterior ribs is seen in 7% of scans and is secondary to _____ .

A: the insertion of the iliocostalis portion of the erector spinae muscles

Q: Increased uptake in the patellae, the "hot" patellae sign, is usually due to _____ .

A: degenerative disease

Q: Lower cervical activity as a normal variant may be secondary to _____ .

A: lordosis, thyroid cartilage uptake, or free ^{99m}Tc-pertechnetate in the thyroid gland

Q: Free TcO_4 from breakdown of tag will localize to the _____ .

A: thyroid gland and gastrointestinal (GI) tract

Q: Colloid formation during tracer preparation will show activity in the _____ .

A: reticuloendothelial system

Q: Aluminum contamination during preparation of the radiopharmaceutical results in _____ .

A: pulmonary activity

Q: True/false: A circular skeletal lesion is more likely benign than malignant.

A: true

Q: The uptake of phosphate bone agents is determined by bony metabolic activity, blood flow, and _____ .

A: sympathetic tone

Q: Loss of _____ leads to an inability to close capillaries. The resultant increase in blood flow causes increased tracer accumulation, as seen in patients with stroke or hemiplegia.

A: sympathetic tone

Q: Hypertrophic osteoarthropathy is most commonly associated with _____ .

A: bronchogenic carcinoma

Q: True/false: Chemotherapy commonly causes decreased kidney uptake.

A: false

Q: In Paget's disease, laboratory findings include increased serum alkaline phosphatase level and elevated serum and urinary _____ levels.

A: hydroxyproline

Q: True/false: Malignant degeneration to sarcoma occurs in 5–10% of patients with Paget's disease.

A: false

Q: Reflux sympathetic distrophy syndrome (RSDS) is also termed _____ .

A: causalgia, Sudeck's atrophy, and shoulder–hand syndrome

Q: Symptoms include _____ .

A: pain, tenderness, vasomotor instability, swelling, and dystrophic skin changes

Q: SPECT has been shown to have an important role in the evaluation of _____ .

A: facial bones, temporomandibular joints, back, and knees

Q: The diphosphonates are characterized by _____ bonds instead of the _____ bonds of phosphates.

A: P-C-P, P-O-P

Q: What are the advantages of diphosphonates over phosphates?

A: They are more stable *in vivo*, have a more rapid blood clearance, and yield a higher bone-to-background ratio than the phosphates

Q: True/false: In a healthy patient, less than 5% of the injected dose of TcMDP remains in the blood 3 hrs after injection.

A: false

Q: Give three findings to support the suspicion for a super scan.

A: very high bone-to-background ratio, absent or faint kidneys, very fast count rate in the axial skeleton

Q: What is the most common neoplastic cause of super scan?

A: Prostatic carcinoma

Q: What is the difference between cold PYP and hot PYP?

A: hot PYP is ^{99m}Tc-labeled pyrophosphate; cold PYP is nonradioactive PYP

Q: When is ^{99m}Tc-PYP used?

A: myocardial infarct avid scan

Q: Why is the cold PYP used for radiolabelling red blood cells?

A: it contains stannous chloride, which is a reducing agent that allows TcRBC tagging

Q: What are the current agents used for bone scanning?

A: methylene diphosphonate (MDP), methylene hydroxydiphosphonate (MHDP)

Q: What are the mechanisms of osseous uptake on bone scan?

A: chemabsorption of apatite crystal and incorporation into immature collagen

Q: Which factors influence the degree of uptake in the bone scan.

A: skeletal blood flow, osteoblastic activity, calcium turnover

Q: Name three mechanisms of extraosseous uptake of bone agent.

A: hyperemia-increased delivery, calcification or ossification-bind with phosphonate, necrosis–calcium influx

Q: What patient factor will reduce the quality of a bone scan?

A: obesity, CHF, renal insufficiency

Q: What is a four-phase bone scan?

A: additional 24-hr delayed images

Q: What is the significance of positive first and second phases but normal third phase?

A: suggests soft tissue process without bone involvement

Q: What is the significance of normal first and second phases but positive third phase?

A: bone lesion that is usually chronic, not hypervascular or active

Q: What is the significance of a positive fourth phase?

A: suggestive of osteomyelitis or malignant tumor rather than arthritis or benign bone disease

Q: When is the 3PBS false-negative?

A: diminished delivery due to vascular disease or occlusion

Q: If the 3PBS is conclusive for osteomyelitis, what is the benefit of also performing a gallium scan?

A: monitoring therapeutic response; a bone scan may remain positive for 1–2 years

Q: What is the scintigraphic pattern of osteomyelitis in children?

A: "hot" focus in metaphyseal region

Q: What is the meaning of photon defect in the area of an active infection?

A: may represent an abscess with necrotic center in advanced osteomyelitis or ischemia associated with early osteomyelitis

Q: What is reflex sympathetic dystrophy?

A: a symptom complex involving the extremities, with pain, hyperesthesis, tenderness, trophic changes and vasomotor instability

Q: What is the scintigraphic finding for RSD?

A: increased flow and diffusely increased periarticular activity in delayed images

Q: What is the explanation for the abnormal bone scan in RSD?

A: loss of sympathetic stimulation results in vasodilatation, increased blood flow, and bone turnover; there is also associated synovitis contributing to the diffusely increased periarticular activity

Q: How does hemiplegia influence RSD?

A: the flow may be decreased due to diminished metabolic demand, but there will be increased periarticular uptake due to RSD

Q: What is the scintigraphic finding for pseudoarthrosis?

A: irregular discrete focal increased uptake at the site of pseudoarthrosis

Q: How do you determine the maturity of MO? Why is this important?

A: serial bone scans showing decreasing or stabilizing activity; immature MO will grow back after surgical excision

Q: What other nuclear medicine procedure can be used for MO evaluation?

A: bone marrow scan using ^{99m}Tc-colloid

Q: Pertaining to the last question, what will the scintigraphic finding be?

A: a mature MO will concentrate radiocolloid, and immature MO may demonstrate little bone marrow activity

Q: What are the agents we use for bone marrow scanning?

A: ^{99m}Tc-albumin colloid, ^{99m}Tc-sulfur colloid, ^{99m}Tc-antimony colloid

Q: What is shin splint?

A: periostitis along the posteromedial angle of the tibia, tear of the tibialis posterior muscle or soleus muscle–tendon complex

Q: How does the scintigraphic appearance of shin splint differ from stress fracture?

A: the lesion extends 50% or more transversely into the cortex

Q: What is the usual scintigraphic appearance of stress fracture?

A: focal rounded uptake

Q: What is the scintigraphic appearance of shin splint?

A: longitudinal wavy irregular uptake in the periosteal aspect of the posteromedial tibia

Q: What is the three phase bone scan finding in acute phase of acute vascular necrosis (AVN)?

A: diminished flow and cold defect in the delayed views

Q: What is the finding in chronic/reparative phase of AVN?

A: increased or normal flow with increased uptake

Q: How is the bone marrow scan used in AVN?

A: a cold defect in the region of increased uptake on bone scan indicates the bone scan abnormality is due to infarct

Q: What is the scintigraphic pattern of septic arthritis in four-phase bone scan?

A: diffusely increased flow and blood pool images in the first and second phase, third phase may be normal or positive, fourth phase normal

Q: What are the scintigraphic findings of cellulitis?

A: increased flow and blood pool images in the first and second phase, third phase may be normal or positive, fourth phase normal

Q: What are possible complications of hip prosthesis?

A: infection, loosening, fracture, heterotopic bone formation, myositis ossificans

Q: How do you evaluate prosthesis problems in nuclear medicine?

A: three-phase bone scan and labelled white cell or gallium scan if needed

Q: What is the scintigraphic finding of loosening of the femoral component?

A: focal skeletal phase uptake at the tip of the hardware

Q: What are the scintigraphic findings of infected femoral component?

A: increased flow and intense uptake around the prosthesis' stem

Q: What does a "discordant" gallium bone scan pattern indicate?

A: acute osteomyelitis

Q: How is radionuclide arthrogram performed?

A: using ^{99m}Tc-albumin colloid in a routine arthrogram procedure

Q: How is this compared to contrast arthrogram?

A: more sensitive to detect loosening

Q: What do you see in a poor tagged ^{99m}Tc-MDP scan?

A: gastric, salivary gland, thyroid uptake

Q: Give at least three differentials of pulmonary uptake in a bone scan.

A: sarcoidosis, diffuse metastases, malignant effusion, radiation, microlithiasis

Q: What are the three most common causes of hepatic uptake in a bone scan?

A: metastases, technical (colloid formation, elevated aluminum impurity), recent liver spleen scan

Q: What are two common causes of splenic uptake on a bone scan?

A: sickle cell anemia, recent liver spleen scan

Q: Name three causes of gastric uptake on a bone scan.

A: free TcO^4, milk-alkali syndrome, hypercalcemia

Q: What is the most common cause of thyroid uptake on a bone scan?

A: free TcO^4

Q: Name three causes of breast uptake on a bone scan.

A: breast CA, gynecomastia, mastitis, normal variant

Q: Give at least three differentials of cardiac uptake in a bone scan.

A: myocardial infarct, cardiac failure, renal failure, pericardial effusion, pericarditis, amyloidosis, inadequate interval between injection and scan

Q: Name three common causes of diffuse calvarial uptake in a bone scan.

A: hyperostosis, marrow expansion, Paget's disease

Q: Name three causes of focal brain uptake in a bone scan.

A: infarct, metastasis, abscess

Q: What is the most common cause of skin activity on a bone scan?

A: urine contamination

Q: Give three differentials of generalized decreased osseous uptake in a bone scan.

A: technical (Al impurity, poor tagging), osteoporosis; obesity

Q: Give five differentials of focally decreased osseous uptake in a bone scan.

A: AVN, radiation, lytic mets, early fracture, bone cyst, early osteomyelitis

Q: Name three primary tumors causing photopenic metastases.

A: renal, thyroid, multiple myeloma, lung

Q: Describe the scintigraphic pattern of Paget's disease.

A: expansile or thickening of the bone with sharp demarcation from the normal area

Q: How does Paget's disease affect bone?

A: increased bone resorption accompanied by increased bone formation

Q: Describe the scintigraphic pattern of multiple myeloma.

A: mostly normal, some may reveal diminished uptake, increased uptake at fracture sites

Q: What is the general scintigraphic characteristic of metabolic bone diseases?

A: diffusely increased bone activity

Q: How do you evaluate amyloidosis with nuclear medicine study?

A: using the classic ^{99m}Tc-(PYP) has a mixed result; better results are obtained with the newer ^{123}I-serum amyloid P component (SAP)

Q: What is the scintigraphic pattern of benign pleural effusion in bone scan?

A: diffusely diminished activity of a portion of the thorax

Q: What is the scintigraphic pattern of malignant pleural effusion in bone scan?

A: increased activity

Q: What is the scintigraphic pattern of radiation osteitis in bone scan?

A: increase activity at first several weeks, followed by defect

Q: What is the scintigraphic pattern of extramedullary hematopoiesis in bone scan?

A: increased uptake, especially in the ribs with paravertebral activity

Q: What is the scintigraphic pattern of early fracture in bone scan?

A: cold defect within the first few hours

Q: What are the possible explanations for this finding?

A: rupture of vascular supply from fracture, too early for reactive bone formation

Q: How soon will a fracture remain positive, and what is its time course in the bone scan?

A: cold defect in the first few hours, then increasing activity up to a few weeks or months, then tapering off until resolved

Q: What is the meaning of persistent "hot" uptake in a remote fracture?

A: nonhealing or nonunion, refracture in the same area

Q: What is the role of ^{89}Sr?

A: ^{89}Sr, an analogue of calcium, is absorbed in the sites of bone mets, where it irradiates the lesion, producing palliation of pain for an average of 6 months after a single dose

Q: What are the radionuclides used for pain palliation in bone metastases?

A: ^{32}P, ^{89}Sr, ^{186}Re, ^{153}Sm

Q: What is the most common side effect?

A: bone marrow suppression

Q: The proportion of bone radiopharmaceutical actually picked up by bone is approximately:
a. 10–15%
b. 30%
c. 50%
d. 75%
e. 90%

A: c

Q: The following neoplasm does not frequently metastasize to bone (as compared to the others):
a. ovary
b. prostate
c. lung
d. lymphoma
e. breast

A: a

Q: The clearance of bone radiopharmaceutical from the blood into the bone's hydroxapatite crystal plateaus at approximately:
a. 5 min
b. 20 min
c. 1 hr
d. 2 hr
e. 3 hr

A: b

Q: Photon deficient bone scan lesions may be found in:
a. metastatic disease
b. Legg-Perthe's disease
c. infarct of sickle cell disease
d. osteomyelitis
e. all of the above

A: e

Q: True/false: Bone scans are more sensitive than radioiodine surveys in detecting metastatic thyroid lesions.

A: false

Q: Which of the following commonly cause photopenic lesions on bone scan?
a. malignant melanoma
b. Ewing's sarcoma
c. multiple myeloma
d. hypernephroma
e. colon carcinoma

A: c, d

Q: The injected material most likely to be associated with increased injection site uptake on a bone scan is:
a. demerol
b. compazine
c. vitamin B_{12}
d. insulin
e. iron dextran

A: e

Q: Super scans are generally associated with:
a. several focal areas of increased uptake
b. absent kidney visualization
c. enhanced salivary gland uptake
d. all of the above
e. none of the above

A: b

Q: Pulmonary, gastric, and enhanced kidney activity on a bone scan is often seen in patients with:
a. myelosclerosis
b. histiocytosis
c. metastases from osteogenic sarcoma
d. hyperparathyroidism
e. hyperthyroidism

A: d

Q: In acute fractures, bone scans in patients under 50 years old first become positive:
a. within 7 hr
b. 48–72 hr
c. 4– days
d. 7–10 days

A: a

Q: Increased uptake of bone tracer in a patient's hemithorax on both anterior and posterior views is most often associated with:
a. postmastectomy state
b. unilateral hyperlucent lung
c. pleural effusion
d. calcific pleuritis

A: c

Q: The *flare phenomenon* in bone scanning is most often reflective of:
a. worsening metastatic disease
b. "healing" response to chemotherapy
c. renewed growth of metastatic lesions following hormonal suppression
d. specific pattern of metastatic disease involving iliac wings

A: b

Q: True/false: The chemical structure of organic phosphates, such as (MDP), includes a phosphate-carbon (P-C-P) linkage.

A: true

Q: True/false: Gallium scans that show lesions that are intense and discordantly smaller in distribution than on bone scans are strongly suggestive of osteomyelitis.

A: true

Match the following five statements with the appropriate radiopharmaceutical:
a. ^{67}Ga citrate
b. ^{111}In WBCs
c. both
d. neither

Q: Best for the more acute infection.

A: b

Q: Has physical half life close to 3 days.

A: c

Q: Can best detect extent of edema associated with osteomyelitis

A: d

Q: Can be studied with a low energy collimator

A: d

Q: Multiple blood transfusions may cause false negative study

A: a

Q: Uptake that starts at the end of a long bone and extends well into the diaphyseal shaft is most typical of:
a. fibrous dysplasia
b. Paget's disease
c. osteomyelitis
d. osteonecrosis

A: b

Q: True/false: Neuropathic (Charcot) joints generally are associated with proximal hyperemia in the involved extremity on bone scan.

A: true

Q: Unilateral increased uptake in a distal extremity on bone scan may be associated with:
a. paralysis of a limb
b. reflex sympathetic dystrophy
c. intra-arterial injection
d. all of the above
e. none of the above

A: d

Q: Liver uptake on a bone scan caused by dystrophic ossification is most often due to:
a. hyperparathyroidism
b. metastatic colon carcinoma
c. hemosiderosis
d. metastatic melanoma
e. hepatoma

A: b

Q: Splenic uptake on a bone scan is most often seen in:
a. cirrhosis with portal hypertension
b. hypersplenism
c. sickle cell disease
d. lymphoma
e. splenic abscess

A: c

5 Cardiac

Q: What intracellular ion does thallium most closely mimic?

A: Potassium

Q: What is the half-life of ^{201}Tl?

A: 73 hr

Q: How does ^{201}Tl decay?

A: electron capture

Q: What element does ^{201}Tl decay to?

A: 201-Mercury

Q: True/false: The photons used for ^{201}Tl imaging come from the decay of ^{201}Tl.

A: False: They come from the decay of ^{201}Hg.

Q: What are the energies and abundances of the photons used for ^{201}Tl imaging?

A: 69–83 keV (95% abundance), 135 keV (3.5% abundance), 167 keV (10% abundance)

Q: What percent of ^{201}Tl entering the coronary circulation is extracted by the myocardium?

A: 88%

Q: What is the relationship between ^{201}Tl extraction by the myocardium and coronary blood flow at physiological flow rates?

A: a linear increase in ^{201}Tl uptake proportional to coronary blood flow

Q: What happens to the extraction efficiency of ^{201}Tl at very high flow rates?

A: it increases

Q: What happens to the extraction efficiency of ^{201}Tl at very low flow rates?

A: it decreases

Q: How much of an injected dose of ^{201}Tl remains in the blood 5 minutes after injection?

A: 5%

Q: When does peak uptake in the myocardium occur after injection of ^{201}Tl?

A: 10–20 minutes

Q: How much of the IV ^{201}Tl dose localizes in the myocardium in a normal patient?

A: 5%

Q: What is the difference between early and delayed ^{201}Tl uptake?

A: early uptake represents blood flow, delayed uptake represents redistribution to equilibrium

Q: What are the two causes of decreased uptake on early ^{201}Tl images?

A: reduced blood flow or absence of viable myocardium (scar)

Q: What is the cause of reduced uptake on delayed ^{201}Tl images?

A: scar

Q: What is the cause of reduced uptake on post-stress images with fill-in on delayed images?

A: myocardial ischemia

Q: What patient preparation is recommended for ^{201}Tl imaging?

A: the patient should ideally be fasting for 4 hours before injection

Q: Why should ^{201}Tl be injected as close as possible to a direct venous injection?

A: to prevent adsorption to IV tubing or to venous structures being exposed to medications

Q: What is the usual initial dose of ^{201}Tl for myocardial imaging?

A: 2.0–3.5 mCi

Q: When is imaging begun after a dose of ^{201}Tl for myocardial imaging?

A: 10 min

Q: What type of collimator is used for ^{201}Tl for planar myocardial imaging?

A: low-energy, high-resolution, or low-energy all-purpose collimator

Q: What views should be obtained for planar imaging of ^{201}Tl for myocardial imaging?

A: 35–40° left anterior oblique, 60–70° left anterior oblique and left lateral

Q: What are the choices for energy windows for imaging of ^{201}Tl for myocardial imaging?

A: a 20–25% asymmetric window centered at 80 keV or a 20% symmetric window centered at 69–83 keV and an optional 20% window centered at 167 keV

Q: What is the advantage of using an asymmetric window centered at 80 keV for ^{201}Tl imaging?

A: this reduces measurement of scattered higher energy K-α ^{201}Hg X rays scattered in the energy range of the lower energy ^{201}Hg K-β X rays

Q: What is the advantage of using a 20% window centered at 167 keV for ^{201}Tl imaging?

A: it will increase the count rate by 10%

Q: How many counts are typically acquired for a planar image with ^{201}Tl myocardial imaging?

A: 300–500K

Q: How much time typically elapses for a planar image with ^{201}Tl myocardial imaging?

A: 8–10 minutes

Q: What type of collimator is used for ^{201}Tl for SPECT myocardial imaging?

A: low-energy, high resolution, or low-energy all-purpose collimator

Q: What are typical details of a SPECT acquisition for ^{201}Tl myocardial imaging?

A: 180° arc from 45° right anterior oblique to 135°left posterior oblique with imaging completed in 20–35 minutes; acquisition details differ among camera systems

Q: What is apical thinning on ^{201}Tl myocardial imaging?

A: physiologically reduced uptake in the apex

Q: What is the appearance of the valve plane on ^{201}Tl myocardial imaging?

A: it appears as a defect in uptake in the anterior and lateral images

Q: What kind of attenuation artifact is commonly seen in women on ^{201}Tl myocardial imaging?

A: anterior wall reductions in uptake due to breast attenuation

Q: What artifact does diaphragmatic attenuation cause on imaging?

A: decreased uptake in the inferior wall

Q: How can diaphragm attenuation be minimized in planar ^{201}Tl myocardial imaging?

A: image the patient in the left lateral decubitus position

Q: What is the meaning of right ventricular uptake on resting planar ^{201}Tl myocardial imaging?

A: right ventricular hypertrophy: the right ventricle is not normally seen on resting planar ^{201}Tl myocardial imaging

Q: What is the only organ that does not take up ^{201}Tl?

A: the brain; thallium does not cross the blood–brain barrier

Q: What organs other than the heart normally accumulate ^{201}Tl?

A: salivary glands, thyroid, skeletal muscle, kidneys

Q: What is the appearance of acute infarctions on ^{201}Tl myocardial images?

A: a cold defect due to absent blood flow and peri-infarct ischemia and edema

Q: What is the sensitivity of ^{201}Tl myocardial imaging for detecting acute myocardial infarction in the immediate postinfarction period (<8 hours)?

A: about 90%

Q: What is the sensitivity of ^{201}Tl myocardial imaging for detecting acute myocardial infarction at 24 hours postinfarction?

A: about 60%

Q: Why is ^{201}Tl myocardial imaging for detecting acute myocardial infarction in the immediate postinfarction period (<8 hours) nonspecific?

A: defects may either be an acute infarction or an old myocardial infarction

Q: How is ^{201}Tl myocardial imaging used for risk stratification and prognosis after myocardial infarction?

A: patients with larger infarcts are at higher risk of mortality

Q: How is ^{201}Tl myocardial imaging used for the assessment of thrombolytic therapy of acute myocardial infarction?

A: pre- and post-thrombolysis images can be used to determine the degree of reperfusion

Q: What is *stunned myocardium*?

A: injured myocardium that is distal to a lysed thrombus that has normal ^{201}Tl uptake but is akinetic on wall motion studies

Q: What is *hibernating myocardium*?

A: chronically ischemic myocardium that is viable but appears cold on immediate ^{201}Tl images and is akinetic on wall motion studies

Q: What is the rationale of using exercise in ^{201}Tl myocardial perfusion imaging?

A: normal coronary arteries dilate during exercise and flow increases, while stenotic vessels do not dilate and flow does not increase to the same degree as in normal myocardium

Q: How do you calculate maximum predicted heart rate?

A: 220-age in (bpm)

Q: What percent of maximal predicted heart rate is considered an adequate stress test?

A: 85%

Q: How do you calculate the double product of an exercise stress test?

A: maximum systolic blood pressure × maximum heart rate

Q: What is the most common reason for a false-negative ^{201}Tl stress test?

A: failure to exercise adequately

Q: What should be done with cardiac drugs before a ^{201}Tl stress test?

A: they should be stopped at the discretion of the patient's attending

Q: What medications interfere with cardiac stress testing, and how long should they be stopped?

A: β blockers (72 hr), calcium channel blockers (48–72 hr), and long-acting nitrates (12 hr)

Q: How long should patients continue to exercise after injection of ^{201}Tl for a stress myocardial perfusion study?

A: 30–90 sec

Q: How long should patients wait between injections of ^{201}Tl for a stress myocardial perfusion study? Why not longer and why not shorter?

A: 10 min; longer periods may miss rapid redistribution; shorter periods cause "cardiac creep" artifact

Q: How do planar stress ^{201}Tl myocardial images differ from rest images?

A: on the stress images, the target-to-background ratio is higher, right ventricular activity is commonly seen on the stress images, and less activity is seen in the liver and abdominal structures

Q: What is the meaning of normal ^{201}Tl myocardial uptake on rest and post-stress images?

A: normal myocardium

Q: What is the meaning of reduced ^{201}Tl myocardial uptake on the post-stress images and normal uptake on the rest images?

A: ischemic myocardium

Q: What is the meaning of reduced ^{201}Tl myocardial uptake on the post-stress images and improved uptake on the rest images?

A: ischemic myocardium, possibly with scar

Q: What is the meaning of reduced ^{201}Tl myocardial uptake on the post-stress images and the same uptake on the rest images?

A: scar

Q: What three items should be described for myocardial perfusion defects?

A: location, size, and possible vascular distribution

Q: What is the meaning of reduced ^{201}Tl myocardial uptake on the rest images and the same uptake on the post-stress images?

A: reverse redistribution

Q: What areas of the myocardium are served by the left anterior descending coronary artery?

A: the anterior wall and septum

Q: What areas of the myocardium are served by the left circumflex coronary artery?

A: the lateral and posterior walls

Q: What areas of the myocardium are served by the right coronary artery?

A: the inferior wall, the inferior septum, and the right ventricle

Q: What two findings, other than myocardial defects, should be described on ^{201}Tl myocardial perfusion imaging?

A: left ventricular dilation and pulmonary uptake

Q: What is the upper limit of normal for the quantitative lung-to-heart ratio on ^{201}Tl myocardial perfusion imaging?

A: 0.5

Q: What are the possible causes of increased lung uptake on ^{201}Tl myocardial perfusion imaging?

A: left ventricular dysfunction, severe coronary artery disease, and heavy smoking

Q: What is bulls-eye analysis of ^{201}Tl myocardial perfusion imaging?

A: a quantitative presentation of myocardial uptake and washout

Q: Why is the specificity of ^{201}Tl myocardial perfusion imaging difficult to measure?

A: only patients with positive or equivocal myocardial perfusion imaging are sent for cardiac catheterization

Q: What is the sensitivity of ^{201}Tl myocardial perfusion imaging for the detection of coronary artery disease among patients without a previous history of coronary artery disease who exercise adequately?

A: 80–85%

Q: How is ^{201}Tl myocardial perfusion imaging used to manage the patient with an acute myocardial infarction?

A: patients with a single fixed defect are given medical therapy; all others are considered for more invasive evaluation and therapy, as they are at higher risk for subsequent cardiac events and death

Q: How is ^{201}Tl myocardial perfusion imaging used to assess the patient with a previous coronary artery bypass or angioplasty?

A: successful revascularization results in no areas of ischemia; scars will not be affected by revascularization; and perioperative infarction of an ischemic area will appear as a fixed defect

Q: What is the rationale for reinjection of ^{201}Tl before delayed myocardial perfusion imaging?

A: 15–35% of ischemia segments do not fill in or normalize by 4–5 hr

Q: What are the alternatives to exercise for performing stress ^{201}Tl myocardial perfusion imaging?

A: dipyridamole and adenosine

Q: How much can dipyridamole and adenosine increase coronary blood flow?

A: fourfold to fivefold

Q: What enzyme does dipyridamole inhibit?

A: adenosine deaminase

Q: What is the main advantage of adenosine over dipyridamole?

A: adenosine has a shorter plasma half-life

Q: What are the main symptoms and side effects of adenosine and dipyridamole?

A: chest pain, nausea, vomiting, dizziness, headache, shortness of breath, hypotension

Q: What is the antidote to dipyridamole?

A: aminophylline 125–250 mg IV

Q: What additional patient preparation is required for patients undergoing stress testing with adenosine or dipyridamole?

A: patients must be off methylxanthines (like theophylline) and caffeine

Q: Where in the myocardial cell does ^{99m}Tc-sestamibi localize?

A: the mitochondrion.

Q: How does the myocardial extraction of ^{99m}Tc-sestamibi compare with 201Tl?

A: at resting flows the extraction fraction of 99mTc-sestamibi is about half that of 201Tl and decreases with increasing flow

Q: How much of a dose of ^{99m}Tc-sestamibi remains in the blood at 10 min after injection?

A: about 5%

Q: What is the clearance time of ^{99m}Tc-sestamibi from the myocardium?

A: 5 hr

Q: Why should ^{99m}Tc-sestamibi myocardial imaging be delayed at least 30 min after injection?

A: to allow for clearance of tracer from the lungs and liver

Q: How is ^{99m}Tc-sestamibi excreted?

A: by hepatobiliary and renal routes

Q: What is the usual time between injection of and myocardial imaging?

A: 30–90 min

Q: What is the usual dose of ^{99m}Tc-sestamibi for myocardial perfusion imaging?

A: 10–30 mCi

Q: For planar ^{99m}Tc-sestamibi for myocardial perfusion imaging, what kind of collimator is typically used?

A: low-energy, high-resolution

Q: For planar ^{99m}Tc-sestamibi for myocardial perfusion imaging, how many counts are typically obtained for each image?

A: 750–1000 K

Q: What two types of additional myocardial imaging can be performed with ^{99m}Tc-sestamibi but not with ^{201}Tl?

A: gated SPECT and first-pass radionuclide angiography

Q: What is the advantage of performing gated SPECT and first-pass radionuclide angiography with ^{99m}Tc-sestamibi myocardial perfusion imaging?

A: both ventricular function and myocardial perfusion can be assessed with a single dose of the radiopharmaceutical

Q: What doses of ^{99m}Tc-sestamibi are used for a one-day rest/stress myocardial perfusion imaging protocol?

A: about 8 mCi for rest imaging followed by 22 mCi for stress imaging

Q: What doses of ^{99m}Tc-sestamibi are used for a two-day rest/stress or stress/rest myocardial perfusion imaging protocol?

A: about 22 mCi for both rest and stress imaging

Q: How do the diagnostic criteria for infarction and ischemia differ between ^{201}Tl and ^{99m}Tc-sestamibi?

A: they do not differ

Q: What is the difference between first-pass study cardiac ventriculography and equilibrium cardiac ventriculography?

A: in first-pass studies, all data collection occurs during the initial transit of tracer through the heart: in equilibrium studies, data are collected over many cardiac cycles using the tracer that remains in the blood pool

Q: What is the radiopharmaceutical of choice for equilibrium gated blood pool imaging?

A: ^{99m}Tc-labeled RBCs

Q: What are the names of the three different methods for labeling RBCs with ^{99m}Tc?

A: *in vivo*, modified *in vivo*, and *in vitro*

Q: How is *in vivo* labeling of RBCs with ^{99m}Tc performed?

A: the patient is injected with cold stannous pyrophosphate; 15 to 30 min later, the patient is injected with ^{99m}Tc-pertechnetate

Q: Where in the RBC does ^{99m}Tc bind?

A: to the β chain of hemoglobin

Q: What is the labeling yield of *in vivo* method for labeling RBCs with ^{99m}Tc?

A: about 80% and as low as 60–65%

Q: What are five causes of poor *in vivo* RBC labeling?

A: drug interactions, circulating antibodies, incorrect amount of stannous ion, excess carrier ^{99m}Tc, inappropriate procedure

Q: What are six drugs that can cause poor *in vivo* RBC labeling?

A: heparin, iodinated contrast media, doxyrubicin, methyldopa, hydralazine, quinidine

Q: How can poor labeling of RBCs be detected?

A: excessive gastric, thyroid, and soft tissue uptake

Q: How is modified *in vivo* labeling of RBCs with ^{99m}Tc performed?

A: the patient is injected with cold stannous pyrophosphate; 15 to 30 minutes later, 3–5 ml of blood are withdrawn into an anticoagulated syringe containing ^{99m}Tc-pertechnetate; the syringe is incubated for 10 min; the patient is injected with the contents of the syringe

Q: What is the labeling yield of modified *in vivo* method for labeling RBCs with ^{99m}Tc?

A: about 90%

Q: How is *in vitro* labeling of RBCs with ^{99m}Tc performed?

A: blood is withdrawn into an anticoagulated syringe; the blood is added to a reaction vial containing stannous chloride; after incubation, sodium hypochlorite is added to the vial to oxidize extracellular stannous ion; ^{99m}Tc-pertechnetate is added to the vial and incubated; the patient is injected with the contents of the vial

Q: What is the labeling yield of the *in vitro* method for labeling RBC with ^{99m}Tc?

A: about 95% or greater

Q: What non-red cell agent is available for equilibrium-gated blood pool imaging?

A: ^{99m}Tc-human serum albumin

Q: What is the advantage of ^{99m}Tc-human serum albumin over ^{99m}Tc-labeled RBCs for equilibrium-gated blood pool imaging?

A: ^{99m}Tc-human serum albumin can be prepared more rapidly

Q: What is the disadvantage of ^{99m}Tc-human serum albumin over ^{99m}Tc-labeled RBCs for equilibrium-gated blood pool imaging?

A: ^{99m}Tc-human serum albumin has more liver uptake and had less blood pool activity

Q: What is the main difference in the pharmacokinetics of ^{99m}Tc-labeled RBCs and ^{99m}Tc-human serum albumin?

A: ^{99m}Tc-labeled RBCs circulate with an effective half-life close to 6 hr, while ^{99m}Tc-human serum albumin leaks into the interstitium with a half-life of 4 hr

Q: What is the critical organ and dose for IV ^{99m}Tc-labeled RBCs?

A: the spleen, 0.11 rad/mCi

Q: What agents may be used for first-pass imaging?

A: any red blood cell agent, ^{99m}Tc-DTPA, ^{99m}Tc-pertechnetate, ^{99m}Tc-sulfur colloid, or almost any other ^{99m}Tc agent

Q: What kind of IV injection is required for a first-pass radionuclide angiogram?

A: the injection must be in a compact bolus

Q: Which vein of the arm is preferred for injection for a first-pass radionuclide angiogram?

A: a medial vein in the basilic system in the antecubital fossa; the cephalic veins should be avoided

Q: How many frames per sec should be obtained for a first-pass radionuclide angiogram?

A: 15–30

Q: How much data acquisition time is typically required for a first-pass radionuclide angiogram?

A: 30 sec

Q: In what situation should the data acquisition time for a first-pass radionuclide angiogram be increased?

A: congestive heart failure

Q: What is the best camera position for assessing right and left ventricular function during a first-pass radionuclide angiogram?

A: a 20° right anterior oblique to separate the atria from the ventricles

Q: What are two advantages of first-pass radionuclide angiography over equilibrium-gated blood pool imaging?

A: acquisition time is short, allowing imaging at peak stress; right ventricular ejection fraction can be measured

Q: What is the major disadvantage of first-pass radionuclide angiography over equilibrium-gated blood pool imaging?

A: low counting statistics

Q: What is used as the gating signal for equilibrium-gated blood pool imaging?

A: the R wave of the electrocardiogram

Q: How many frames are obtained for a typical equilibrium-gated blood pool imaging?

A: 16–24 frames

Q: What is the typical duration of a frame in equilibrium-gated blood pool imaging?

A: about 40–50 msec

Q: What is the advantage and disadvantage of increasing the number of frames in equilibrium-gated blood pool imaging?

A: more frames increase temporal resolution, but counting statistics in each individual frame are reduced

Q: How many cardiac cycles are acquired in a typical equilibrium-gated blood pool imaging study?

A: 100–300 cycles

Q: How many counts are acquired per image in a typical equilibrium-gated blood pool imaging study?

A: 250K counts

Q: How do dysrhythmias affect the quality of an equilibrium-gated blood pool imaging study?

A: they degrade the study because segments of cardiac cycle that are added together do not correspond

Q: What (ECG) patterns on a rhythm strip will degrade an equilibrium-gated blood pool imaging study?

A: atrial fibrillation with an irregular ventricular response, skeletal muscle activity, giant T waves, pacemaker artifacts

Q: What two computer techniques can be used to limit the problem of dysrhythmias degrading an equilibrium-gated blood pool imaging study?

A: filtering data from premature contractions and postextrasystolic beats and list mode acquisition

Q: What views are typically obtained for a resting equilibrium-gated blood pool imaging study?

A: A 10° right posterior oblique, a 30–60° left anterior oblique, and a left posterior oblique

Q: How should one determine the angulation for a left anterior oblique image for an equilibrium-gated blood pool imaging study?

A: adjust the angle until the left and right ventricles are maximally separated

Q: What are the common features of protocols for exercise radionuclide ventriculography?

A: one image is taken at rest, and at least one other image is taken during peak stress

Q: How does one assess wall motion on a radionuclide ventriculogram?

A: observe the study in a repetitive cine loop and look for shrinkage of the ventricle at its periphery and thickening of the septum

Q: What is akinesis?

A: absence of ventricular contraction

Q: What is hypokinesis?

A: reduced ventricular contraction

Q: What is dyskinesis?

A: outward ventricular movement during contraction

Q: What is tardokinesis?

A: ventricular contraction that is present, but delayed in timing

Q: What walls of the left ventricle have the greatest excursion?

A: the free wall and apex

Q: What is the typical wall motion appearance of myocardial scar?

A: akinesis or hypokinesis

Q: What is the typical wall motion appearance of myocardial ischemia?

A: akinesis or hypokinesis

Q: Qualitative analysis of a radionuclide angiogram should assess what four features?

A: cardiac chamber size, regional wall motion, overall biventricular performance, extracardiac abnormalities

Q: What is the principle assumption underlying the measurement of left ventricular ejection fraction on a radionuclide ventriculogram?

A: the activity from the heart is directly proportional to ventricular volume

Q: Which frame of a radionuclide ventriculogram is the end-systolic frame?

A: the frame with the fewest counts in the left ventricular region of interest

Q: Which frame of a radionuclide ventriculogram is the end-diastolic frame?

A: the frame with the greatest counts in the left ventricular region of interest

Q: What is the formula for the left ventricular ejection fraction on a radionuclide ventriculogram?

A: ejection fraction = (end diastolic counts − end systolic counts)/(end diastolic counts − background counts)

Q: What is the usual range for a normal left ventricular ejection fraction measured by a radionuclide ventriculogram?

A: 0.55–0.75

Q: Why do the trailing frames of a radionuclide ventriculogram have fewer counts?

A: because of slight variations in the length of the cardiac cycle

Q: What is a cause of a large fall-off in the counts on trailing frames of a radionuclide ventriculogram?

A: wide variation of cardiac cycle length, as in atrial fibrillation

Q: How does the computer create Fourier phase and amplitude images from a radionuclide ventriculogram?

A: each pixel over time is fit to a sine wave of a particular amplitude and phase

Q: What does the amplitude image of a Fourier analysis of a radionuclide ventriculogram represent?

A: the maximum count variation for each pixel

Q: What does the phase image of a Fourier analysis of a radionuclide ventriculogram represent?

A: the time delay from the R wave to the start of the cardiac cycle for each pixel

Q: How do wall motion abnormalities appear on amplitude images of a Fourier analysis of a radionuclide ventriculogram?

A: reduced amplitude

Q: How does dyskinesia appear on phase images of a Fourier analysis of a radionuclide ventriculogram?

A: opposite phase to the ventricles

Q: How does Wolff-Parkinson-White syndrome appear on phase images of a Fourier analysis of a radionuclide ventriculogram?

A: affected areas are slightly out of phase to the remainder of the ventricle

Q: How does the computer create a stroke volume image from a radionuclide ventriculogram?

A: subtract the end-systolic image from the end-diastolic image

Q: How does the computer create an ejection fraction image from a radionuclide ventriculogram?

A: subtract the end-systolic image from the end-diastolic image and divide the difference by the end-diastolic image

Q: What is the appearance of akinesia on an ejection fraction image?

A: reduced intensity

Q: How does the computer create a paradox image from a radionuclide ventriculogram?

A: subtract the end-diastolic image from the end-systolic image

Q: What is the appearance of dyskinesia on a paradox image?

A: increased intensity

Q: What is the hallmark of an acute myocardial infarction on a radionuclide ventriculogram?

A: regional wall motion abnormality at the site of the infarction and a decrease in global ejection fraction

Q: True/false: Reduced ejection fraction indicates the presence of congestive heart failure.

A: false

Q: What percent of patients with acute myocardial infarctions have abnormal ejection fractions?

A: 75%

Q: How is a radionuclide ventriculogram helpful prognostically in patients with acute myocardial infarction?

A: the lower the ejection fraction, the worse the prognosis, and worsening ejection fraction over time indicates worsening prognosis

Q: What type of infarction is associated with right ventricular wall motion abnormalities?

A: inferior wall infarctions

Q: What is the hallmark of ischemia on exercise radionuclide ventriculogram?

A: failure of the ejection fraction to increase with stress and development of wall motion abnormalities not present at rest

Q: What are the two major limitations of the exercise radionuclide ventriculogram for assessing myocardial ischemia?

A: difficulty of getting patients to achieve and maintain maximal stress during imaging and nonspecificity of an abnormal response

Q: What is the sensitivity of the exercise radionuclide ventriculogram for assessing myocardial ischemia among patients who exercise adequately?

A: 85–94%

Q: In clinical practice, what is the specificity of the exercise radionuclide ventriculogram for assessing myocardial ischemia among patients who exercise adequately?

A: 55%

Q: What six conditions other than coronary artery disease can cause an abnormal response to stress on a radionuclide ventriculogram?

A: cardiomyopathy, myocarditis, valvular heart disease, pericardial disease, drug toxicity, prior surgery or injury

Q: How is radionuclide ventriculography useful in the follow-up of patients undergoing coronary artery bypass grafting?

A: improvement of global ejection fraction and regional wall motion document the success of surgical intervention

Q: How is radionuclide ventriculography useful in the follow-up of patients with valvular heart disease?

A: one can measure ejection fraction and ventricular size at rest and stress; one can also measure stroke volume ratios to look for regurgitation

Q: What is the typical radionuclide ventriculogram appearance of patients with congestive cardiomyopathies?

A: the ventricle is dilated with global diffuse hypokinesia and a low ejection fraction

Q: What segments can be spared in the wall motion abnormalities of a patient with congestive cardiomyopathies?

A: the basal and septal segments

Q: How is radionuclide ventriculography useful in the follow-up of patients undergoing cardiotoxic chemotherapy?

A: patients can be followed and the drug discontinued if there is a drop of ejection fraction of more than 15%

Q: How is radionuclide ventriculography useful in the follow-up of patients with pulmonary disease?

A: the radionuclide ventriculogram can differentiate between cor pulmonale and left-sided heart disease

Q: How can left-to-right shunt be measured with a first-pass radionuclide angiogram?

A: one can detect early recirculation into the pulmonary circuit

Q: How can right-to-left shunt of congenital heart disease be measured with scintigraphy?

A: one can inject ^{99m}Tc-macroaggregated albumin (MAA) and measure the ratio of activity over the lung and the brain

Q: How is ^{82}Rb made?

A: from a strontium/rubidium generator

Q: How is ^{13}N ammonia made?

A: in a cyclotron

Q: How is ^{18}FDG made?

A: in a cyclotron

Q: What is the positron emitter ^{82}Rb a marker of in myocardial imaging?

A: myocardial blood flow

Q: What is the positron emitter ^{13}N ammonia a marker of in myocardial imaging?

A: myocardial blood flow

Q: What is the positron emitter ^{18}FDG a marker of in myocardial imaging?

A: myocardial glucose metabolism

Q: The findings of a PET scan with ^{82}Rb or ^{13}N ammonia are most similar to a SPECT scan with what agent?

A: ^{201}Tl or ^{99m}Tc-sestamibi

Q: Under normal conditions, what percent of the heart's energy needs are met through glucose metabolism?

A: 15%

Q: What is the preferred metabolic substrate of ischemic myocardium?

A: glucose

Q: What is the typical ^{82}Rb/^{18}FDG PET scan pattern of normal myocardium?

A: normal blood flow (normal ^{82}Rb uptake) with normal glucose metabolism (normal ^{18}FDG uptake)

Q: What is the typical ^{82}Rb/^{18}FDG PET scan pattern of ischemic myocardium?

A: reduced blood flow (decreased ^{82}Rb uptake) with normal glucose metabolism (normal ^{18}FDG uptake)

Q: What is the typical ^{82}Rb/^{18}FDG PET scan pattern of scarred myocardium?

A: reduced blood flow (decreased ^{82}Rb uptake) with reduced glucose metabolism (reduced ^{18}FDG uptake)

Q: What agent is available to perform myocardial infarct avid imaging?

A: ^{99m}Tc-pyrophosphate

Q: Why does ^{99m}Tc-pyrophosphate localize in myocardial infarctions?

A: infarcted tissue has an influx of calcium with the formation of calcium-phosphate complexes; the tracer diffuses into the cell and binds to these complexes

Q: When is the optimum time for myocardial infarct imaging with ^{99m}Tc-pyrophosphate?

A: 24–48 hr

Q: What is the usual dose of ^{99m}Tc-pyrophosphate for myocardial infarct imaging?

A: 15–25 mCi

Q: What is the reason for a ring or donut pattern of uptake with myocardial infarct imaging with ^{99m}Tc-pyrophosphate?

A: the edges of the infarct with residual blood flow show uptake of tracer, while the central part of the infarct has no uptake because there is no blood flow to deliver the tracer

Q: What is the usual time delay between injection of ^{99m}Tc-pyrophosphate and imaging for a myocardial infarct?

A: 3–4 hr

Q: What structures in the chest normally localize ^{99m}Tc-pyrophosphate?

A: the skeletal structures: ribs, sternum, spine

Q: How soon does a myocardial infarct become positive with ^{99m}Tc-pyrophosphate imaging?

A: 12 hr

Q: When is myocardial infarct uptake maximal with ^{99m}Tc-pyrophosphate imaging?

A: 2–3 days

Q: How long does it take for myocardial infarct uptake of ^{99m}Tc-pyrophosphate to return to normal?

A: 14 days

Q: What is the minimal mass of a myocardial infarction that can be detected with ^{99m}Tc-pyrophosphate imaging?

A: 3 g

Q: What is the sensitivity of ^{99m}Tc-pyrophosphate imaging for transmural myocardial infarctions?

A: 95%

Q: What is the sensitivity of ^{99m}Tc-pyrophosphate imaging for subendocardial myocardial infarctions?

A: 65%

Q: What is the specificity of ^{99m}Tc-pyrophosphate imaging for myocardial infarctions?

A: 90%

Q: What are four causes of false-positive focal myocardial uptake on ^{99m}Tc-pyrophosphate imaging?

A: old myocardial infarction with persistent uptake, calcification, ventricular aneurysm, costal cartilage calcification

Q: What are seven causes of false-positive diffuse myocardial uptake on ^{99m}Tc-pyrophosphate imaging?

A: myocardial, pericarditis, cardiomyopathy, amyloidosis, radiation therapy, cardiotoxic chemotherapy, blood pool activity

Q: What is the prognostic significance of ^{99m}Tc-pyrophosphate uptake for more than 3 months?

A: such patients are at high risk for future myocardial infarctions

Q: What is the usual clinical situation in which ^{99m}Tc-pyrophosphate uptake is ordered to detect myocardial infarction?

A: when all other routine tests, such as history, physical exam, ECG, and serum enzymes, are nondiagnostic

Q: "The lights dim, then fade to black. The curtain is about to rise. It's the most electric moment at the theater—that instant of darkness just before the show begins. It is called . . ."

A: a) *Beforia*
  b) *Curtension*
  c) *Operahension*
  d) *Expectricity*
  e) *Un-curtainty*

Q: Since thallium, sestamibi, and teboroxime are rapidly cleared from the blood and concentrated by the myocardium, their regional distribution is generally proportional to _____ .

A: blood flow

Q: Thallium is extracted by the blood as a _____ analogue through the mechanism of _____ by the Na-K ATP pump.

A: K$^+$, active transport

Q: Sestamibi is extracted by _____ across mitochondria and plasma membranes.

A: passive diffusion

Q: Thallium is produced in a _____ .

A: cyclotron

Q: The purpose of thallium reinjection is to increase the _____ of **stress/redistribution** thallium imaging in detecting viable myocardium.

A: sensitivity

Q: Compared to normal myocardium, thallium washes out of ischemic myocardium at a(n) _____ rate.

A: slower

Q: Compared to normal myocardium, thallium washes out of infarcted myocardium at a(n) _____ rate.

A: equal

Q: Which cardiac perfusion agent washes out at a faster rate, thallium or sestamibi?

A: thallium

Q: With which cardiac perfusion agent is redistribution the key parameter in detecting reversible ischemia, thallium or sestamibi?

A: thallium

Q: Due to the effects of redistribution, the distribution of thallium on delayed images corresponds to the distribution of _____ .

A: viable tissue

Q: In exercise stress sestamibi imaging, sestamibi is injected at _____ and exercise is continued for 2 more min.

A: peak exercise

Q: The critical organ for thallium is the _____ while that for ^{99m}Tc-sestamibi and ^{99m}Tc-teboroxime is the _____ .

A: kidney, proximal colon

Q: Dipyridamole causes _____ of normal coronary vessels.

A: dilatation

Q: Dipyridamole administration results in the accumulation of _____ .

A: adenosine

Q: The patient's heart rate _____ and the blood pressure _____ in response to dipyridamole.

A: increases, decreases

Q: Blood flow to myocardium supplied by normal coronary vessels will _____ in response to dipyridamole, while blood flow to myocardium supplied by significantly narrowed vessels will _____ or, on occasion, _____ in response to dipyridamole.

A: increase, not change, decrease

Q: Dipyridamole is contraindicated in patients with asthma because of its ability to induce _____ .

A: bronchospasm

Q: If bronchospasm or significant ischemia occurs during dipyridamole infusion, _____ should be administrated to reverse these effects.

A: aminophylline

Q: In SPECT imaging compared to planar imaging, the sensitivity is _____ but the specificity is _____ .

A: higher, lower

Q: Planar and SPECT thallium imaging are most sensitive in detecting disease in the distribution of the _____ artery and least sensitive in detecting disease in the distribution of the _____ artery.

A: left anterior descending (LAD), circumflex

Q: Transient dilation of the left ventricle on an exercise stress image compared to a rest image signifies _____ .

A: left ventricular dysfunction

Q: Dipyridamole is administered intravenously at a dose of _____ for a total of _____ min.

A: .142 mg/kg/min, 4

Q: On planar thallium imaging, the septum, supplied by the _____ , is best seen on the _____ view.

A: left anterior descending artery, left anterior oblique (LAO)

Q: On planar thallium imaging, the posterobasal wall of the left ventricle, supplied by the _____ is best seen in the _____ view.

A: left circumflex artery, steep (70°) LAO

Q: On planar thallium imaging, the anterolateral wall of the left ventricle, supplied by the _____ artery is best seen on the _____ view.

A: left anterior descending, anterior

Q: On planar thallium imaging, the inferior wall of the left ventricle, supplied by the _____ artery is best seen on the _____ view.

A: right coronary, anterior

Q: On planar thallium imaging, the apex of the left ventricle, supplied by either the _____ artery or the _____ artery, depending on dominance, is best evaluated in the _____ and _____ view.

A: left circumflex, right coronary, anterior, steep (70°) LAO

Q: On planar thallium imaging, the anterior wall of the left ventricle, supplied by the _____ artery is best evaluated on the _____ view.

A: left anterior descending, steep (70°) LAO

Q: In SPECT cardiac imaging the apex is best evaluated on the _____ and _____ views.

A: horizontal long axis, vertical long axis

Q: In SPECT cardiac imaging the anterior wall is best evaluated on the _____ and _____ views.

A: short axis, vertical long axis

Q: In SPECT cardiac imaging the septum is best evaluated on the _____ and _____ views.

A: short axis, horizontal long axis

Q: In SPECT cardiac imaging the lateral wall is best evaluated on the _____ and _____ views.

A: short axis, horizontal long axis

Q: In SPECT cardiac imaging the inferior wall is best evaluated on the _____ and _____ views.

A: short axis, vertical long axis

Q: List four nonpathologic causes of defects on SPECT cardiac imaging.

A: breast or diaphragmatic attenuation, patient motion, incorrect long axis selection during processing, recent meal

Q: List three nonfixed coronary causes of defects in SPECT myocardial perfusion imaging.

A: vasospasm, myocardial bridge, left bundle branch block

Q: List four noncoronary cardiac disease entities that cause defects on SPECT cardiac imaging.

A: aortic stenosis, aortic insufficiency, dilated cardiomyopathy, hypertensive cardiomyopathy

Q: On a gated blood pool study, overestimating background activity results in a falsely _____ left ventricular ejection fraction.

A: elevated

Q: Since right ventricular end diastolic volume is greater than left ventricular end diastolic volume, the right ventricular ejection fraction is expected to be _____ than the left ventricular ejection fraction.

A: lower

Q: Including a portion of the left atrium in the region of interest of the left ventricle at end-systole will result in an ejection fraction that is falsely _____ .

A: decreased

Q: "You pull up to a red light, and in the car next to you, you notice a man. His windows are rolled up, so no sound escapes. But obviously the radio is on full blast, because this fellow is rocking and writhing and pounding the steering wheel while he mouths the words. This silent but oh-so-active tableau is called . . ."

A: a) *Autoerockicism*
   b) *Park 'n' Roll*
   c) *Brake Dancing*
   d) *Vehicular Hummicide*
   e) *Carrythmia*
   f) *Traffic Jamming*

Q: A new approach to detecting infarcted myocardium involves the _____ labelling of monoclonal antibodies to _____ .

A: ^{111}In, cardiac myosin

Q: In gated blood pool imaging a photopenic halo surrounding all the chambers is indicative of a _____ .

A: pericardial effusion

Q: On gated blood pool imaging a photopenic zone surrounding the left ventricle is suggestive of _____ .

A: left ventricular hypertrophy

Q: In order to optimize the target-to-background ratio in antimyosin imaging the ideal time for imaging is _____ after injection.

A: 48–72 hrs

Q: On gated blood pool imaging, paradoxical systolic motion of a focal region of the left ventricular wall suggests the presence of a(n) _____ .

A: aneurysm

Q: A gated blood pool scan or myocardial perfusion scan may show larger and more severe abnormalities in the acute phase of a myocardial infarct compared to several weeks later due to the phenomenon of myocardial _____ .

A: stunning

Q: A fixed area of decreased uptake on a stress/redistribution thallium scan can be caused by:
a. myocardial infarct
b. "hibernating myocardium"
c. normal anatomic thinning
d. a and c
e. all of the above

A: e

Q: All of the following have been used as pharmacologic stress agents in association with myocardial perfusion imaging except:
a. dobutamine
b. furosemide
c. dipyridamole
d. adenosine

A: b

Q: A 70-year-old male undergoing a modified Bruce treadmill stress protocol has a target heart rate of:
a. 160
b. 150
c. 128
d. 120

A: c

Q: True/false: A stress study followed in several hours by a rest study is the protocol of choice for sestamibi myocardial perfusing imaging.

A: false

Q: The sensitivity for detecting myocardial ischemia is clearly greater on sestamibi as compared to thallium studies.

A: false

Match the following four statements with the appropriate radiopharmaceutical:
a. ^{201}Tl chloride
b. ^{99m}Tc-sestamibi
c. ^{99m}Tc-teboroxime
d. a and b
e. a, b and c

Q: Most rapid washout from heart

A: c

Q: Redistribution from a single injection characteristic of ischemia

A: a

Q: A fixed defect on stress/rest imaging can represent hibernating myocardium, i.e., severe ischemia

A: e

Q: Serendipitous detection of mediastinal parathyroid adenoma possible

A: d

Q: Decreased inferior wall uptake on a myocardial perfusion scan may be caused by:
a. myocardial ischemia
b. diaphragmatic attenuation
c. myocardial infarct
d. all of the above
e. none of the above

A: d

Q: Hibernating myocardium may be best confirmed on:
a. reinjection redistribution thallium images
b. rest/stress sestimibi study
c. 24-hour delayed thallium images
d. ^{18}F-FDG PET scan

A: d

Q: Diminished septal activity on a stress myocardial perfusion study may be seen as an expected finding in:
a. mitral stenosis
b. Wolff-Parkinson-White syndrome
c. left bundle branch block
d. all of the above
e. none of the above

A: c

Q: The earliest indicator of congestive heart failure is a drop in:
a. left ventricular ejection fraction
b. left ventricular stroke volume
c. cardiac output
d. pulse pressure

A: a

Q: The most common indication for performing resting multigated acquisition (MUGA) cardiac studies is:
a. cardiac injury following catheterization
b. adriamycin toxicity
c. detection of coronary artery disease
d. detection of valvular heart disease

A: b

Q: True/false: Intracardiac shunts may be detected on perfusion lung scan.

A: true

Q: True/false: Intracardiac shunts may be detected on first pass radionuclide angiograms.

A: true

Q: True/false: Intracardiac shunts may be detected on MUGA cardiac studies.

A: false

Q: During normal aerobic metabolism the primary substrate used by the heart for energy is/are _____ .

A: fatty acid

Q: Ischemic myocardium will show _____ uptake of ^{18}F labelled F-FDG.

A: increased

Q: With respect to PET imaging of the heart, ^{82}Rb (rubidium) is used to measure myocardial _____ .

A: perfusion

Q: True/false: Published reports support an approximately 95% sensitivity and specificity of PET myocardial perfusion studies for diagnosing coronary artery disease.

A: true

Q: True/false: Ischemic myocardium, relative to normal myocardium, has:

increased perfusion	**A:** false
increased fatty acid metabolism	**A:** false
increased glucose metabolism	**A:** true
hyperkinetic wall motion	**A:** false

Q: True/false: The percent stenosis of a coronary artery is the sole determinant of the significance of coronary artery diseases.   **A:** false

Q: True/false: PET studies demonstrate considerably higher sensitivities for coronary artery disease detection than those utilizing SPECT.   **A:** false

Q: True/false: PET studies demonstrate considerably higher specificities for coronary artery disease detection than those utilizing SPECT.   **A:** true

Q: Evaluation of coronary artery disease by PET-FDG studies in patients with diabetes mellitus is linked by their _____ .   **A:** altered glucose metabolism

6 Central Nervous System

Q: What is the physiologic principle behind blood–brain barrier imaging?

A: tracers stay within the blood pool and diffuse into the brain only when the blood–brain barrier is disrupted

Q: What three tracers are used for blood–brain barrier imaging?

A: ^{99m}Tc-pertechnetate, ^{99m}Tc-DTPA, and ^{99m}Tc-glucoheptanate

Q: What is the main disadvantage of ^{99m}Tc-pertechnetate for blood–brain barrier imaging?

A: it localizes physiologically in the choroid plexus

Q: Why does ^{99m}Tc-glucoheptanate have better uptake in brain tumors than other blood–brain barrier imaging agents?

A: as a glucose analog it may serve as a substrate for tumor metabolism

Q: How do corticosteroids affect blood–brain barrier imaging?

A: they may diminish uptake because corticosteroids decrease blood–brain barrier permeability

Q: How is blood–brain barrier imaging performed?

A: blood flow images are taken every 2–3 sec for one minute, then 750K count immediate static images are taken in multiple views, then, 1.5–2 hours later, 750K count delayed static images are obtained in multiple views

Q: On blood–brain barrier imaging, how much uptake is present in the normal brain?

A: none

Q: What structures are seen normally on blood–brain barrier imaging?

A: the scalp and venous sinuses

Q: What are the findings of subdural hematoma on blood–brain barrier imaging?

A: peripherally reduced flow on dynamic images with increased uptake on delayed images

Q: What are the findings of a ventriculitis on blood–brain barrier imaging?

A: bilaterally increased uptake in the region of the lateral ventricles

Q: What are the findings of an abscess on blood–brain barrier imaging?

A: a focal area of increased uptake on delayed imaging with a cold center developing as the abscess progresses

Q: What are the findings of herpes encephalitis on blood–brain barrier imaging?

A: increased flow and uptake in the affected temporal lobe

Q: What is the characteristic finding of an infarct on the angiogram portion of a blood–brain barrier scan?

A: reduced early perfusion with increased delayed perfusion–the "flip-flop" phenomena

Q: How long after an infarct is the "flip-flop" perfusion first seen on blood–brain barrier imaging?

A: in the first few days

Q: What is "luxury perfusion"?

A: increased blood flow to an infarction due to uncoupling of metabolism; typically seen about 5 days after an infarction

Q: What is the best tracer to use to diagnose venous sinus thrombosis?

A: ^{99m}Tc-RBCs

Q: What is the typical finding of venous sinus thrombosis on ^{99m}Tc-RBC imaging?

A: abrupt termination of the midportion of sinus

Q: What are the findings of an arteriovenous malformation on brain imaging with ^{99m}Tc-RBCs?

A: intense uptake on delayed images

Q: What is the advantage of radionuclide angiography over (EEG) in confirming brain death?

A: radionuclide angiography remains accurate in the face of hypothermia and drug intoxication

Q: What are the scintigraphic criteria for brain death on a radionuclide angiogram?

A: presence of a good carotid bolus without intracranial arterial flow

Q: What is the significance of faint visualization of the venous sagittal sinus or transverse sinus on radionuclide angiography to confirm brain death?

A: it may be seen in 10–20% of patients with brain death and does not preclude the diagnosis of brain death as long as there is no intracranial arterial flow

Q: What are the common features of tracers for imaging regional cerebral perfusion?

A: they are small, neutral lipophilic molecules; they rapidly diffuse across the blood–brain barrier; they have high brain extraction and fraction; they remain fixed in the brain

Q: What three tracers are available for cerebral perfusion scintigraphy?

A: ^{123}I-isopropyl iodo-amphetamine (IMP), ^{99m}Tc-hexamethyl propylene amine oxime (HMPAO), and ^{99m}Tc-ethyl cysteine dimer (ECD)

Q: What percentage of a dose of ^{123}I-IMP localizes in the normal brain?

A: 6–9%

Q: What is the usual administered dose of ^{123}I-IMP?

A: 3–6 mCi

Q: What is the main difference between ^{123}I-IMP and ^{99m}Tc-HMPAO in brain uptake and distribution?

A: ^{123}I-IMP demonstrates redistribution that is independent of brain–blood flow

Q: What is the ratio of gray-to-white matter uptake with ^{123}I-IMP?

A: 3–4:1

Q: What percentage of a dose of ^{99m}Tc-HMPAO localizes in the normal brain?

A: 3.5–7%

Q: What is the ratio of gray-to-white matter uptake with ^{99m}Tc-HMPAO?

A: 2.5:1

Q: How do images of ^{123}I-IMP and ^{99m}Tc-HMPAO differ when imaging infarction?

A: ^{123}I-IMP always shows a flow defect, ^{99m}Tc-HMPAO may show luxury perfusion with increased uptake

Q: How long after injection of ^{99m}Tc-HMPAO does peak brain uptake occur?

A: 2 min

Q: What percentage of a dose of ^{99m}Tc-ECD localizes in the normal brain?

A: 6–7%

Q: How long after injection of ^{99m}Tc-ECD does peak brain uptake occur?

A: 2 min

Q: How do ^{99m}Tc-HMPAO and ^{99m}Tc-ECD differ in terms of blood pool clearance?

A: blood pool clearance is faster with ^{99m}Tc-ECD

Q: How do the circumstances of injection affect cerebral perfusion imaging?

A: stimulation (e.g. visual, auditory) during the injection can cause areas of increased uptake in the sites stimulated

Q: What type of image acquisition is required for cerebral perfusion imaging?

A: SPECT acquisition

Q: What is the normal cerebral blood flow in an adult?

A: about 50 ml / min / 100 g

Q: What is the normal cerebral blood flow in a 3- to 10-year-old child?

A: about 100 ml / min / 100 g

Q: How does blood flow change in the occipital lobes when the eyes are open versus closed?

A: about 30% increase

Q: How does an ictal seizure focus affect regional cerebral blood flow?

A: it causes an increase in blood flow

Q: What methods are available to practically quantify absolute regional cerebral blood flow with SPECT?

A: none

Q: What methods are available to quantify absolute regional cerebral blood flow with radionuclide imaging?

A: PET imaging with ^{15}O water or ^{15}C carbon dioxide or ^{133}Xe imaging with a multiprobe detector

Q: What is the critical organ and its radiation dose for ^{123}I-IMP?

A: the lung with 0.84 rads / 6 mCi

Q: What is the critical organ and its radiation dose for ^{99m}Tc-HMPAO?

A: the lacrimal glands with 5.2 rads / 20 mCi

Q: How long after infarction will decreased blood flow be seen on a cerebral perfusion scan?

A: immediately

Q: In patients with cerebral infarcts why are defects on cerebral perfusion imaging often larger than on CT scan?

A: the area of infarction is surrounded by an ischemia area of decreased blood flow

Q: What is the cause of crossed cerebellar diaschisis?

A: increased activity in the cerebellum contralateral to a cerebral infarction is due to increased blood flow to the cerebellum after a loss of suppressive neural activity from the contralateral cortex

Q: What two factors decrease the sensitivity of cerebral perfusion imaging for infarctions?

A: luxury perfusion and difficulty detecting lacunar infarcts

Q: True / false: 180° acquisitions on ^{99m}Tc-HMPAO studies are diagnostically comparable to 360°acquisitions.

A: false

Q: What is the typical scintigraphic pattern of Alzheimer's disease on cerebral perfusion imaging?

A: bilateral posterior temporal and parietal hypoperfusion

Q: What is the typical scintigraphic pattern of Pick's disease on cerebral perfusion imaging?

A: bilateral frontal hypoperfusion

Q: What is the typical scintigraphic pattern of multi-infarct dementia on cerebral perfusion imaging?

A: multiple asymmetric perfusion defects involving both the cortex and deep structures

Q: What is the positive predictive value of brain perfusion scintigraphy for Alzheimer's disease?

A: about 80%

Q: What is the typical scintigraphic pattern of depression on cerebral perfusion imaging?

A: normal perfusion

Q: What is the typical scintigraphic pattern of metabolic brain dysfunction on cerebral perfusion imaging?

A: normal perfusion

Q: What is the typical scintigraphic pattern of Huntington's chorea on cerebral perfusion imaging?

A: reduced perfusion of the caudate

Q: What is the typical scintigraphic pattern of AIDS dementia on cerebral perfusion imaging?

A: multifocal or patchy cortical and subcortical regions of hypoperfusion

Q: What is the typical scintigraphic pattern of an interictal seizure focus on cerebral perfusion imaging?

A: hypoperfusion

Q: What is the typical scintigraphic pattern of an ictal seizure focus on cerebral perfusion imaging?

A: hyperperfusion

Q: What is the sensitivity of brain perfusion SPECT for the detection of interictal seizure foci?

A: about 65–75%

Q: What is the relative sensitivity of brain perfusion SPECT for the detection of ictal versus interictal seizure foci?

A: the sensitivity is greater for ictal foci

Q: How is brain perfusion SPECT useful in conjunction with the Wada test?

A: brain perfusion SPECT can demonstrate the exact territory perfused by the pentobarbital

Q: How is ^{201}Tl imaging useful for the assessment of brain tumors?

A: the degree of ^{201}Tl uptake is proportional to the malignant grade of the tumor, and uptake in the brain distinguishes recurrent brain tumor from radiation necrosis

Q: How is ^{201}Tl imaging useful for the assessment of AIDS patients with intracerebral mass lesions?

A: ^{201}Tl uptake indicates the presence of a brain tumor such as lymphoma; absence of ^{201}Tl uptake indicates the presence of infection such as toxoplasmosis

Q: What tracer is currently used for radionuclide cisternography?

A: intrathecal ^{111}In-DTPA

Q: What is the critical organ and its radiation dose for intrathecal ^{111}In-DTPA?

A: the surface of the spinal cord with 5.0 rads / 0.5 mCi

Q: How can radionuclide cisternography distinguish normal pressure hydrocephalus from cerebral atrophy?

A: cisternography will show prolonged ventricular uptake in normal pressure hydrocephalus

Q: How is radionuclide cisternography used for the detection of cerebrospinal fluid (CSF) leaks?

A: images specifically to look for leaked radioactivity; pledgets placed in the nasal cavity and counted for leaked radioactivity

Q: "For months, you've been too busy to get your 2-year-old a haircut—and it shows. He's all boy, but he's starting to look like *a* late 1960s rock singer. You take him to the park. Sure enough, a fellow parent meanders over and asks, "What's your little girl's name?" This phenomenon is called . . ."

A: a) *Missonderstanding*
   b) *Insexurity*
   c) *Mane Streaming*
   d) *Unboycoming*
   e) *Dysexia*
   f) *Feminine Mystaque*

Q: True/false: In the initial stage of cerebral ischemia regional cerebral blood flow (rCBF) increases.

A: false

Q: True/false: In the initial stage of cerebral ischemia regional oxygen extraction fraction (rOEF) increases.

A: true

Q: True/false: With cerebral infarction, rOEF increases.

A: false

Q: True/false: With cerebral infarction, cerebral metabolic rate for glucose (CMRglc) increases.

A: false

Q: True/false: Following cerebral infarction, local cerebral blood flow (LCBF) increases.

A: true

Q: The phenomenon of metabolic changes in the brain distal to the location of ischemic injury is called _____ .

A: diaschisis

Q: In Alzheimer's disease, symmetric decreases in perfusion and metabolism occur in the:
a. frontal lobes
b. brain stem
c. posterior-parietal lobe
d. temporo-parietal region

A: d

Q: True/false: In Parkinson's disease, PET perfusion studies demonstrate decreased perfusion to the basal ganglia contralateral to the affected limb.

A: false

Q: Perfusion and metabolism in seizure foci _____ during the ictal phase and _____ during the interictal phase.

A: increase, decrease

Q: True/false: In Parkinson's disease, there is increased ^{18}F-fluorodopa uptake by the striatum (caudate and putamen nuclei).

A: false

Q: True/false: Concerning brain tumors, an advantage of PET is that it can image metabolically active cells versus gadolinium-enhanced MRI and contrast-enhanced CT, which image areas where there is blood–brain barrier breakdown.

A: true

Q: Under usual conditions, the primary substrate for brain metabolism is:
a. glucose
b. fatty acids
c. proteins
d. none of the above
e. all of the above

A: a

Match the following six causes of dementia with the patterns of cerebral perfusion and/or glucose metabolism with which they are most often associated:
a. decreased glucose metabolism and perfusion in caudate nucleus and putamen
b. hypoperfusion and metabolism in temporoparietal regions
c. severe depression of lenticular nuclei glucose metabolism
d. generalized cortical hypoperfusion and hypometabolism favoring prefrontal regions
e. diffuse hypometabolism affecting sub-cortical more than cortical grey matter
f. scattered foci of decreased cortical perfusion and metabolism
g. decreased perfusion and metabolism uniform across all basal ganglia

Q: Pick's disease   **A:** d

Q: multi-infarct dementia   **A:** f

Q: Alzheimer's disease   **A:** b

Q: Huntington's disease   **A:** a

Q: Wilson's disease   **A:** c

Q: AIDS dementia   **A:** e

Q: True/false: Gadolinium-enhanced MRI and ^{18}F-FDG PET imaging are equally capable of distinguishing between recurrent brain tumor and radiation necrosis.

A: false

Q: True/false: All malignant brain tumors demonstrate hypermetabolism of ^{18}F-FDG.

A: false

Q: True/false: ^{11}C-labelled amino acid analogues may demonstrate hypermetabolism in brain neoplasms that do not show hypermetabolism of ^{18}F-FDG.

A: true

Q: True/false: In differentiating between infectious and neoplastic brain lesions, the presence of hypermetabolism is not useful.

A: false

Q: Which of the following components of a two-headed gamma camera system is not necessary in coincidence detection?
a. crystals
b. PMTs
c. collimators
d. computer
e. all of the above

A: c

Q: True/false: With respect to coincidence detection, in comparison to SPECT imaging, increasing crystal thickness will improve sensitivity of the camera.

A: true

Q: True/false: Positron emitters, for example F-18-FDG, can only be imaged with PET scanners or two-headed gamma cameras.

A: false

Q: Bismuth germinate (BGO) crystals are preferred for PET imaging over sodium iodide (NaI) because:
a. they have better energy resolution
b. they are more efficient scintillators
c. they are more sensitive to 511-keV photons
d. all of the above

A: c

Q: Which of the following PET imaging agents does not measure perfusion?
a. $^{82}RbCl$
b. $^{15}O\text{-}H_2O$
c. $^{13}N\text{-}NH_3$
d. $^{18}F\text{-}FDG$

A: d

Q: Concerning PET versus SPECT imaging, which of the following statements is *not* true?
a. PET is inferior for quantification
b. PET imaging agents are generally of short half-lives
c. PET is more sensitive
d. PET has better spatial resolution
e. attenuation correction is possible with PET

A: a

Q: True/false: The positron emitter ^{15}O can be administered via IV injection or inhalation.

A: true

Q: True/false: SPECT radiopharmaceuticals are cheaper to produce because
most do not require an on-site cyclotron.

A: true

Q: True/false: Attenuation correction is
more accurate for SPECT since only one
photon is attenuated versus two for
positron emitters.

A: false

Q: True/false: PET has more uniform
resolution and higher sensitivity.

A: true

Q: True/false: Many useful single photon
emitters have stable biologic counterparts
that can be used to label compounds of
biologic interest.

A: false

True/false: PET studies of the brain have
been used for in-vivo quantification of:

Q: Glucose utilization

A: true

Q: Blood flow

A: true

Q: Blood volume

A: true

Q: CSF volume

A: false

Q: CSF production rates

A: false

Q: Blood–brain barrier integrity

A: true

Q: Receptor sites

A: true

Q: The brain almost exclusively uses
_____ as its substrate for energy.

A: glucose

Q: True/false: ^{18}F-FDG freely crosses the
blood–brain barrier via the same carrier-
mediated transport system as glucose.

A: true

Q: With respect to PET imaging of the
brain, the term *CMRGlc* refers to
_____ .

A: cerebral metabolic rate of glucose

Q: True/false: The normal global CMRGlc
based on studies in normal healthy
volunteers is approximately 30 μmol
glucose.mm/100 g brain.

A: true

Q: True/false: Local cerebral metabolic
rates of glucose (specific areas of the brain
such as the thalamus, basal ganglia, lobes)
can be determined through PET studies.

A: true

Q: The major limitation on being able to
determine local cerebral metabolic rates of
glucose by PET studies is the
_____ .

A: size of the area of interest

Q: True/false: Approximately 20–30 mCi of ^{18}F-FDG should be administered for a brain study.

A: false

Q: True/false: A routine FDG study can be performed 5 min after radiopharmaceutical administration.

A: false

Q: True/false: External stimuli can increase regional glucose metabolism within particular areas of the brain.

A: true

Q: Hypometabolism in the thalamus ipsilateral to an infarcted basal ganglia demonstrates the phenomenon of _____ .

A: diaschisis

Q: The phenomenon of high blood flow in areas of the brain involved by nonacute infarction is termed _____ .

A: luxury perfusion

Q: Because of areas of the brain involved by nonacute infarction demonstrate relative hyperperfusion compared to their oxygen requirements, the oxygen extraction fraction (OEF) in these regions _____ .

A: decreases

Q: True/false: PET studies show that in the immediate postinfarct period some patients demonstrate increased OEF in the involved region of the brain. This indicates that in these patients, flow would be adequate to meet local metabolic demands.

A: false

Q: Patients with Alzheimer's disease demonstrate the greatest decrease in metabolism in the _____ cortex.

A: parietal

Q: True/false: Global glucose metabolism compared to normals decreases to a greater degree in multi-infarct dementia than in Alzheimer's dementia.

A: false

Q: True/false: Small white matter lacunar infarcts are much more easily identified with PET-^{18}F-FDG studies than by CT.

A: false

Q: True/false: CT can reliably distinguish Alzheimer's from multi-infarct dementia.

A: false

Q: True/false: In Huntington's disease, changes in the caudate nuclei can be observed on PET earlier than with CT.

A: true

Q: Cerebral glucose metabolism and cerebral blood flow are _____ during seizures.

A: increased

Q: Cerebral glucose metabolism and cerebral blood are _____ in the postinfarct period.

A: decreased

True / false: Medicare reimbursement is currently available for PET studies used to:

Q: detect lung cancer

A: false

Q: identify seizure foci in patients with new onset epilepsy and no other workups

A: false

Q: diagnose congenital heart disease

A: false

Q: distinguish residual brain tumor from fibrotic tissue

A: true

Q: identify seizure foci in patients refractory to drug therapy

A: true

Q: Planar brain scintigraphy has a resolution of approximately _____ at the brain's surface. Multiple detector SPECT cameras are able to distinguish lesions as small as _____ , while PET can differentiate structures as small as _____ in size.

A: 1 cm, 8 mm, 5 mm

Q: ^{99m}Tc-pertechnetate, ^{99m}Tc-glucoheptonate, and ^{99m}Tc-DTPA are all examples of _____ markers.

A: extracellular fluid

Q: Extracellular fluid markers are normally excluded from cerebral tissue by the _____ .

A: blood–brain barrier

Q: Pertechnetate is loosely bound to _____ , and is slowly cleared from the bloodstream.

A: albumin

Q: Uptake of radiotracer by the choroid plexus makes _____ a less desirable radiopharmaceutical for dynamic brain flow imaging than TcDTPA or Tc-labelled RBCs.

A: ^{99m}Tc-pertechnetate

Q: If ^{99m}Tc-pertechnetate is to be used in brain flow scintigraphy, the patient should be given _____ to block the choroid plexus.

A: potassium perchlorate

Q: The typical adult dose of potassium perchlorate is _____ . Children between the ages of 2 and 12 should receive _____ , while infants under the age of 2 should be given _____ .

A: 200 mg, 100 mg, 50 mg

Q: _____ is a neoplasm that accumulates excessive amounts of pertechnetate.

A: choroid plexus papilloma

Q: Tracers used to measure cerebral blood flow must have a high _____ extraction fraction.

A: first pass

Q: When evaluating for brain death, a tourniquet may be placed around the patient's head to exclude activity from the _____ circulation.

A: external carotid

Q: EEG tracings are unreliable for determining brain death in patients with _____ or _____ .

A: barbiturate poisoning, hypothermia

Q: Brain flow scintigraphy as a test for brain death is unaffected by _____ or _____ .

A: barbiturate intoxication, body temperature

Q: The "hot nose" sign may be seen in brain death and is due to increased flow in the _____ circulation.

A: external carotid

Q: According to the recent literature, faint visualization of the _____ in the absence of arterial flow is consistent with brain death.

A: superior sagittal sinus

Q: Areas of breakdown in the blood–brain barrier appear as foci of _____ uptake when extracellular fluid markers are used.

A: increased

Q: ^{99m}Tc-HMPAO and ^{123}I-IMP are lipophilic tracers that differ from extracellular fluid markers due to their ability to cross the _____ .

A: blood–brain barrier

Q: ^{99m}Tc-HMPAO and ^{123}I-IMP are taken up by the brain in proportion to _____ .

A: regional blood flow

Q: ^{99m}Tc-HMPAO binds intracellularly and reaches equilibrium in _____ .

A: 5 min

Q: ^{123}I-IMP reaches equilibrium in _____ , but redistributes over several hours.

A: 20 min

Q: True/false: Persistent ventricular filling on a radionuclide cisternogram is diagnostic of communicating hydrocephalus.

A: true

Q: The major advantage of ^{99m}Tc-HMPAO over ^{123}I-IMP is its significantly better _____ .

A: resolution

Q: In the determination of brain death, one of the advantages of ^{99m}Tc-HMPAO over ^{123}I-IMP is its ability to evaluate the _____ .

A: posterior fossa

Q: ^{123}I-IMP and thallium show evidence of _____ in the brain and heart, respectively.

A: redistribution

Q: The _____ sign has been described in stroke patients and is due to slower collateral circulation to infarcted parenchyma.

A: "flip-flop"

Q: ^{123}I has a _____ half-life, which limits the availability of ^{123}I-IMP for emergency studies.

A: 13-hr

Q: Epileptic seizure foci typically show increased uptake of ^{99m}Tc-HMPAO and ^{123}I-IMP during the _____ phase and decreased uptake during the _____ period.

A: ictal, interictal

Q: In a normal ^{99m}Tc-HMPAO study, greatest uptake of activity is seen in _____ matter structures.

A: grey

Q: A _____ collimator tilted at 30° allows a SPECT detector to remain close to the patient's head and clear the shoulders.

A: slant hole

Q: A normal SPECT study cannot exclude multi-infarct dementia, since _____ are often too small to be detected.

A: lacunar infarcts

Q: When compared to SPECT, CT and MRI tend to _____ the extent of cerebral infarction.

A: underestimate

Q: Alzheimer's disease is characterized by symmetric perfusion deficits in the _____ regions on brain SPECT imaging.

A: posterior temporal and parietal

Q: Patients with Huntington's disease show _____ striatal metabolism.

A: decreased

Q: SPECT and PET scans in patients with Parkinson's disease show _____ perfusion to the contralateral basal ganglia.

A: increased

Q: ^{15}O is a _____ emitter with a half-life of 2 min.

A: positron

Q: ^{13}N is PET agent with a half-life of _____ .

A: 10 min

Q: _____ is cyclotron produced and has a half-life of 20 min.

A: ^{11}C

Q: Tomographic imaging can be performed when PET tracers are labeled with _____ .

A: fluorine 18

Q: _____ is used to measure local cerebral metabolic rate.

A: ^{18}F-deoxyglucose (^{18}FDG)

Q: Following transport from the vascular space into brain parenchyma, FDG is phosphorylated by _____ to FDG-6-P04.

A: hexokinase

Q: Diminished temporoparietal uptake of ^{18}FDG is typically seen in _____ .

A: Alzheimer's disease

Q: SPECT and PET studies have both shown decreased rCBF in the _____ lobes of schizophrenics.

A: frontal

Q: In patients with astrocytomas, PET-FDG studies have shown a linear correlation between glucose metabolic rate and _____ .

A: histologic grade

Q: Cerebral blood _____ can be measured using ^{11}C- or ^{15}O-labeled carbon monoxide.

A: volume

Q: Radiolabeled benzamide, lisuride, and spiperone derivatives attach to _____ receptors in the brain.

A: dopamine D-2

Q: Labeled benzapine derivatives attach to _____ receptors in patients with psychotic and movement disorders.

A: dopamine D-1

Q: ^{11}C-labeled _____ is a high-affinity opiate agonist that binds to mu receptors in the central nervous system.

A: carfentanil

Q: _____ is the radiopharmaceutical most frequently used to assess the patency of a V/P shunt.

A: ^{99m}Tc-DTPA

Q: Due to its relatively long half-life, _____ is the preferred radiotracer for nuclear cisternography.

A: ^{111}In-DTPA

Q: Radiotracer normally clears from the basal cisterns and ascends over the convexities by _____ hr postinjection.

A: 24

Q: At 48 hr, all activity should be at the vertex for resorption into the _____ .

A: arachnoid granulations

Q: In nuclear cisternography, radiotracer normally doesn't enter the _____ .

A: lateral ventricles, nasal cavity, internal auditory canal

Q: In _____ hydrocephalus, radiotracer preferentially enters the lateral ventricles.

A: normal pressure

Q: The nasal cavity is packed with _____ when looking for CSF rhinorrhea.

A: pledgets

Q: "You arrive at the doctor's office right on the dot. The receptionist tells you that he'll be right with you. But *National Geographic* gives way to *Newsweek* and *People*, and your name still hasn't been called. Half of you wants to stalk out. The other half knows that if you do, the receptionist will call your name 30 seconds later. This indecision is called . . ."

A: a) *Paradocs*
b) *Indocision*
c) *Docotomy*
d) *Outpatience*
e) *Roomateasim*
f) *Medipause*

Q: Intensity of thallium uptake in primary brain tumors is related to _____ .

A: histologic grade

Q: Thallium uptake does not depend upon breakdown of the blood–brain barrier. Rather, it is due to _____ across the cell membrane, which is increased in malignant tissues.

A: active transport

Q: _____ brain tumor imaging is superior to MRI in distinguishing between recurrent tumor and edema or gliosis.

A: thallium

Q: Thallium brain imaging is useful in distinguishing _____ from _____ in HIV-positive patients.

A: toxoplasmosis, lymphoma

Q: Patients with _____ encephalitis may show abnormal radiotracer uptake in the temporal lobes before positive findings are seen on CT.

A: herpes simplex

Q: A peripheral, crescent-shaped area of increased Tc-DTPA uptake best describes a _____ .

A: subdural hematoma

Match the following six statements with the appropriate brain radiopharmaceutical:
a. ^{123}I-IMP
b. ^{99m}Tc-HMPAO
c. ^{99m}Tc-DTPA
d. all of the above
e. none of the above

Q: does not normally cross the blood–brain barrier

A: c

Q: "redistributes" over several hours.

A: a

Q: requires preparation with oral perchlorate to block unwanted choroid plexus uptake.

A: e

Q: can be used to establish the presence of brain death.

A: d

Q: subacute stroke appears as an area of increased uptake.

A: c

Q: static study is generally performed one hour or longer after injection.

A: c

Q: The most characteristic pattern suggesting Alzheimer's disease on a functional brain scan is:
a. symmetric decrease in frontal lobe perfusion
b. asymmetric basal ganglia uptake
c. symmetric decrease in anteroparietal perfusion
d. symmetric decrease in posterior parietotemporal perfusion

A: d

Q: Intraictal findings in focal seizure disorders on a functional brain scan may include:
a. localized area of increased uptake
b. localized area of decreased uptake
c. a wider area of decreased perfusion than would be predicted from the clinical symptomatology
d. decreased perfusion in the thalamic region

A: a

Q: The amount of injected dose of ^{99m}Tc-HMPAO (Ceretec) that actually localizes in the brain is:
a. 4–6%
b. 10–15%
c. 20–25%
d. 40–50%

A: a

Q: True/false: Abnormal findings on ^{99m}Tc-HMPAO SPECT images in seizure patients generally parallel findings on ^{18}F-FDG PET studies.

A: true

Q: SPECT functional brain imaging has contributed to patient management in:
a. transient ischemia attacks (TIA)
b. epilepsy
c. cocaine abuse
d. all of the above
e. a and b

A: d

Q: Following lumbar subarachnoid instillation of a radiopharmaceutical, the normal time to visualize the activity around the convexity of the brain would be:
a. 4 hr
b. 12 hr
c. 24 hr
d. 48 hr

A: c

Q: The current agent of choice for radionuclide cisternography is:
a. ^{99m}Tc human serum albumin
b. ^{111}In chloride
c. ^{99m}Tc-DTPA
d. ^{111}In-DTPA

A: d

Q: True/false: Persistent ventricular filling and delayed transit around the brain convexity on a radionuclide cisternogram is consistent with normal pressure hydrocephalus.

A: true

Q: True/false: Abnormal findings on ^{99m}Tc-HMPAO SPECT images in seizure patients generally parallel findings on ^{18}F-FDG PET studies.

A: true

7 Endocrine

Q: What is the main difference between how the thyroid handles iodine and pertechnetate?

A: the thyroid organifies iodine, but not technetium

Q: What are three disadvantages to using ^{131}I for thyroid imaging?

A: ^{131}I emits a βparticle, has a high gamma energy, and has a long half-life; these factors combine to result in a high radiation dose to the thyroid

Q: What are the main contaminants of commercial ^{123}I?

A: ^{124}I and ^{125}I; these contaminants increase the radiation dose

Q: Name three advantages of ^{99m}Tc-pertechnetate over ^{123}I for thyroid imaging.

A: cost, convenience (one patient visit), availability

Q: What percentage of a dose of radioiodine is taken up by the thyroid of a euthyroid individual at 24 hrs after dosing?

A: 10–30%

Q: What percent of a dose of ^{99m}Tc-pertechnetate is taken up by the thyroid of a euthyroid individual at 20 minutes after dosing?

A: 0.5–3.5%

Q: How long does nursing need to be stopped for diagnostic doses of ^{123}I?

A: several days

Q: How long does nursing need to be stopped for diagnostic doses of ^{99m}Tc-pertechnetate?

A: 1–2 days

Q: How long does nursing need to be stopped for uptake doses (<30 μCi) of ^{131}I?

A: weeks to months

Q: When does the fetal thyroid begin to concentrate iodine?

A: at 12 weeks of gestation

Q: How does exogenous iodine affect thyroid uptake of radioiodine?

A: exogenous iodine suppress thyroid uptake of radioiodine

Q: What is the dose of ^{99m}Tc-pertechnetate for thyroid imaging?

A: 1–10 mCi

Q: What is the usual time between injection of ^{99m}Tc-pertechnetate and imaging?

A: 20 min.

Q: What is the usual collimator used for ^{99m}Tc-pertechnetate thyroid imaging?

A: a pinhole or high-resolution parallel

Q: What views are typically obtained for ^{99m}Tc-pertechnetate thyroid imaging?

A: anterior and 45° left and right anterior obliques

Q: How many counts are obtained for ^{99m}Tc-pertechnetate thyroid imaging?

A: 200,000–250,000

Q: What route is used to administer radioiodine?

A: oral

Q: What is the dose of ^{123}I for thyroid imaging?

A: 100–400 µCi

Q: What is the usual time between administration of ^{123}I and imaging?

A: 6–24 hrs

Q: What is the usual collimator used for ^{123}I thyroid imaging?

A: a pinhole or high-resolution parallel

Q: What views are typically obtained for ^{123}I thyroid imaging?

A: anterior and 45° left and right anterior obliques

Q: How many counts are obtained for ^{123}I thyroid imaging?

A: 200,000–250,000

Q: What is the dose of ^{131}I for thyroid whole body imaging for thyroid cancer?

A: 2–5 mCi

Q: What is the usual time between administration of ^{131}I for thyroid whole body imaging for thyroid cancer and imaging?

A: 1–3 days

Q: What is the usual collimator used for ^{131}I for thyroid whole body imaging for thyroid cancer?

A: high-energy parallel

Q: What views are typically obtained for ^{131}I for thyroid whole body imaging for thyroid cancer?

A: anterior and posterior chest, abdomen, and pelvis

Q: How much time is used to obtain images for ^{131}I for thyroid whole body imaging for thyroid cancer?

A: 10–20 min per image

Q: How are markers used for thyroid imaging?

A: markers are used to show the location of the sternal notch, chin, thyroid cartilage, and palpable nodules

Q: How much does a normal thyroid gland weigh?

A: 15–20 g

Q: What is the usual length and breadth of a normal thyroid gland?

A: 4–5 cm by 1.5–2 cm

Q: What is a pyramidal lobe?

A: functioning thyroid tissue in the thyroglossal duct remnant that arises from the isthmus and extends superiorly just to the left or right of midline

Q: How do you prove that activity on a thyroid scan is in the esophagus?

A: have the patient drink water and the activity will go away

Q: What is the normal pattern of uptake in the thyroid isthmus?

A: the isthmus may show uptake similar to normal thyroid or may be absent

Q: What other glands in the neck other than the thyroid can be visualized on thyroid imaging?

A: the salivary glands

Q: What four features should be described on a thyroid scan?

A: thyroid size, homogeneity, and configuration; identification and description of hot and cold nodules; identification of extrathyroidal activity; correlation of abnormalities with palpation

Q: What is the typical appearance of a benign nontoxic multinodular goiter?

A: inhomogenous uptake with multiple cold areas of varying size

Q: What is the typical appearance of a goiter due to Graves' disease?

A: homogeneously increased uptake

Q: What is the differential diagnosis of a goiter?

A: multinodular goiter, Graves' disease, thyroid cancer, thyroid metastases, thyroiditis

Q: What is the purpose of a thyroid scan in evaluating a patient with a thyroid nodule?

A: to see whether the nodule is single or multiple, hot or cold

Q: What is the risk of cancer in a solitary cold thyroid nodule?

A: 15–40%

Q: What is the risk of cancer in a warm thyroid nodule?

A: it should be considered the same as a cold thyroid nodule

Q: How does a history of head/neck radiation affect the risk of cancer in a solitary cold thyroid nodule?

A: it moderately increases the risk

Q: What is the difference between an autonomous and nonautonomous hot thyroid nodule?

A: autonomous nodules are not under the control of thyroid stimulating hormone (TSH)

Q: What finding on a thyroid scan demonstrates that a hot nodule is autonomous?

A: suppression of the normal thyroid tissue

Q: What percentage of hot nodules are malignant?

A: less than 1%

Q: How can nodules that are hot on ^{99m}Tc-pertechnetate imaging be cold on ^{123}I imaging?

A: some thyroid neoplasms trap pertechnetate, but cannot organify pertechnetate or iodine

Q: What percentage of nodules that are hot on ^{99m}Tc-pertechnetate imaging are cold on ^{123}I imaging?

A: 2–3%

Q: What radiopharmaceutical should be used to image substernal thyroids, and why?

A: ^{131}I has a high gamma energy which is not affected by sternal attenuation

Q: What is the appearance of a sublingual thyroid on thyroid imaging?

A: a single mass of functional tissue at the base of the tongue with no activity within the normal thyroid bed location

Q: What is the appearance of thyroiditis on thyroid imaging?

A: decreased or absent uptake in the affected part of the thyroid

Q: What types of thyroid cancers can be visualized on radioiodine imaging?

A: follicular and papillary carcinomas

Q: What preparation is required for ^{131}I total body imaging for thyroid cancer?

A: thyroid hormone must be withdrawn to increase TSH

Q: How is a thyroid uptake study performed?

A: the patient takes a dose of radioiodine; a probe measures activity in the neck, thigh, shielded neck, and a standard; the background corrected ratio of neck-to-standard counts is the uptake

Q: How is the thyroid uptake test useful in distinguishing thyroiditis from Graves' disease?

A: in thyroiditis, the uptake is abnormally low; in Graves' disease, the uptake is abnormally high

Q: How is ^{131}I used to treat Graves' disease?

A: The patient is given a dose adjusted for gland weight and uptake; alternatively, a standard treatment dose is used

Q: How do therapeutic doses of radioiodine for Graves' disease and toxic multinodular goiter differ?

A: doses for a multinodular goiter need to be higher

Q: What tracer is most commonly used for parathyroid imaging?

A: ^{99m}Tc-sestamibi

Q: What is the typical finding of parathyroid adenomas on parathyroid imaging with ^{99m}Tc-sestamibi?

A: parathyroid adenomas show delayed washout compared to normal thyroid tissue

Q: "You are about to make a phone call, but you discover the phone cord twisted up into a spaghetti-like mess. The best way to untangle the cord is to dangle the receiver just above the floor and let it spin a few times. What is this procedure called?"

A: a) *Ditwistiture*
b) *Disendanglement*
c) *Total recoil*
d) *Ring Around the Caller*
e) *Cordio Pullmonary Resuscitation*
f) *Twistidigitizing*

Q: True/false: Discordant thyroid nodules (as the term is generally used) do not concentrate ^{99m}Tc-pertechnetate.

A: false

Q: True/false: Scintigraphic visualization of a pyramidal lobe in a hyperthyroid patient favors the diagnosis of toxic nodular goiter.

A: false

Q: True/false: The great majority of "cold" thyroid nodules are benign.

A: true

Q: A whole body survey (post-thyroidectomy) for metastatic thyroid Ca is generally performed with what dose of radioiodine?
a. 100 μCi of ^{131}I
b. 1–2 mCi of ^{123}I
c. 1–5 mCi of ^{131}I
d. 10–15 mCi of ^{131}I
e. any of the above is acceptable

A: c

Q: True/false: Papillary adenocarcinoma of the thyroid most commonly spreads hematogenously to bone and lung.

A: false

Q: True/false: The size of the thyroid gland can be estimated quite well on a gamma camera image.

A: false

Q: True/false: Thyroglossal tract cysts often contain thyroid tissue that functions on ^{123}I or ^{99m}Tc-pertechnetate scans.

A: false

Match the five following clinical entities with the most appropriate radiopharmaceutical:
a. ^{111}In-octreoscan
b. ^{131}I-MIBG
c. ^{131}I-iodocholesterol (NP-59)

Q: adrenal cortical adenoma

A: c

Q: pituitary adenoma

A: a

Q: medullary carcinoma of the thyroid

A: a

Q: pheochromocytoma

A: b

Q: carcinoid tumor

A: a

Q: ^{99m}Tc-sestamibi uptake may be found in:
a. parathyroid hyperplasia
b. parathyroid adenoma
c. thyroid adenoma
d. a and b
e. all of the above

A: e

Q: True/false: In performing ^{201}Tl/^{99m}Tc-pertechnetate parathyroid studies, it is best to perform the pertechnetate study first.

A: false

Q: Perchlorate washout test of the thyroid is useful in the diagnosis of:
a. organification defects
b. Plummer's disease
c. lingual thyroid
d. acute thyroiditis

A: a

Q: True/false: An elevated level of thyroid-stimulating immunoglobulin is specific for Graves' disease.

A: true

Q: True/false: Marine-Lenhart syndrome is Graves' disease with cold nodules.

A: true

Q: True/false: The autoimmune nature of Hashimoto's thyroiditis is reflected by high titers of antithyroglubulin and antimicrosomal antibodies and by lymphocytic infiltration of the thyroid.

A: true

Q: True/false: Because of an organification defect in Hashimoto's thyroiditis, the 2- or 4-hr uptake may be elevated in the face of a lower 24-hr uptake.

A: true

Q: After a total thyroidectomy, thyroid replacement is withheld for 6 weeks to allow the TSH level to rise. A TSH level greater than _____ microU/ml should be reached before the ^{131}I whole-body scan is done.

A: 30

Q: The isotope of choice for detecting thyroid carcinoma metastasis is:
a. ^{131}I
b. ^{123}I
c. ^{125}I
d. ^{99m}Tc-pertechnetate

A: a

Q: The thyroid stores T3 and T4 in the follicles as _____ .

A: thyroglobulin

Q: _____ of thyroglobulin releases T3 and T4 into the blood.

A: hydrolysis

Q: When circulating thyroid hormone is low, negative feedback mechanism inducing pituitary (a) increases pituitary synthesis of TSH or (b) suppresses pituitary synthesis of TSH, which in turn decreases iodine trapping, hormonal synthesis, and release by the thyroid.

A: a

Q: Graves' disease is a systemic immunologic process. Almost all of Graves' disease patients have multiple antibodies to _____ .

A: TSH receptors

Q: Ophthalmopathy and skin changes are seen only in _____ and not in other forms of thyrotoxicosis.

A: Graves' disease

Q: Medullary thyroid carcinoma can occur as an isolated lesion or in association with _____ syndrome.

A: multiple endocrine neoplasia

8 Gastrointestinal

Q: What is the usual tracer and dose for radionuclide esophageal transit scintigraphy?

A: 30 µCi of ^{99m}Tc-sulfur colloid

Q: What type of meal is used for radionuclide esophageal transit scintigraphy?

A: a liquid bolus

Q: What is the critical organ and its absorbed dose for oral ^{99m}Tc-sulfur colloid?

A: the large intestine with a dose of 160 mrad / 300 µCi

Q: How are patients prepared for radionuclide esophageal transit scintigraphy?

A: overnight fast

Q: How is a radionuclide esophageal transit scintigraphy performed?

A: the patient lays supine and practices swallowing nonradioactive boluses; the patient then swallows a radioactive bolus, dry swallows at 30 sec, and then swallows a radioactive bolus every 30 sec for 2 min

Q: Why are multiple swallows required for a radionuclide esophageal transit scintigraphy?

A: there is a 25% incidence of "aberrant" swallows; multiple swallows give a more representative result

Q: What is the cause of "abberant" swallows?

A: swallows followed by a dry swallow that inhibits the initial swallow and causes delayed transit

Q: Hoe does one calculate esophageal transit time?

A: the time between the initial entry of the bolus into the esophagus until all but 10% of the initial activity remains.

Q: What esophageal abnormality is radionuclide esophageal scintigraphy most sensitivity for detecting?

A: achalasia

Q: What is the patient preparation for gastroesophageal reflux scintigraphy in adults?

A: overnight fast

Q: What is the radiopharmaceutical, dose and meal used for gastroesophageal reflux scintigraphy in adults?

A: 300 μCi ^{99m}Tc- sulfur colloid in 150 ml of orange juice

Q: What is the patient preparation for gastroesophageal reflux scintigraphy in children?

A: overnight fast

Q: What is the radiopharmaceutical, dose, and meal used for gastroesophageal reflux scintigraphy in children?

A: 5 μCi/kg of ^{99m}Tc-sulfur colloid in 10 ml of water followed by the child's routine meal

Q: What images are obtained for gastroesophageal reflux scintigraphy in children?

A: 5–10 sec dynamic images of the anterior abdomen and chest for 60 minutes and a 2–4 hr delayed image of the chest to look for aspiration.

Q: Why is abdominal compression not used for gastroesophageal reflux scintigraphy in children?

A: it is nonphysiologic and does not increase the detection rate of reflux in children

Q: What three features of reflux should be described in gastroesophageal reflux scintigraphy in children?

A: the height of the reflux in the esophagus, the duration of the reflux, and the time from the meal

Q: What other radionuclide technique can be used for accurately detecting pulmonary aspiration?

A: a radionuclide salivagram where tracer is placed on the tongue and dynamic images are obtained

Q: What are the two functionally distinct areas of the stomach involved in gastric emptying?

A: the fundus and the antrum

Q: What are the common symptoms of delayed gastric emptying?

A: early satiety, bloating, nausea, vomiting

Q: What are the symptoms of rapid gastric emptying?

A: palpitations, diaphoresis, weakness, diarrhea

Q: What is the most common cause of chronic gastroparesis?

A: diabetes

Q: What drugs are used to treat chronic gastroparesis?

A: metoclopramide, domperidone, cisapride, erythromycin

Q: What is the ideal method for radiolabeling chicken liver for a radionuclide gastric emptying study?

A: inject ^{99m}Tc-sulfur colloid intravenously into a live chicken and then sacrifice the chicken

Q: What methods are available for radiolabeling food *in vitro?*

A: inject chicken liver with ^{99m}Tc-sulfur colloid and cook the liver or mix ^{99m}Tc-sulfur colloid with eggs and scramble the eggs

Q: What tracer is used to measure liquid gastric emptying in single isotope studies?

A: ^{99m}Tc-sulfur colloid

Q: What tracer is used to measure liquid gastric emptying in a dual isotope study, simultaneous with solid phase emptying?

A: ^{111}In-DTPA

Q: What characteristics of a meal affect its rate of gastric emptying?

A: liquidity, texture, volume, weight, particle size, caloric density, nutrient composition

Q: When performing gastric emptying sstudies, why must each laboratory follow an established protocol for making a solid phase meal or establish normal values for their meal?

A: the way that the meal is made affects the normal value

Q: What is the advantage of dual isotope gastric emptying studies over solid phase studies?

A: there is little advantage; solid phase is all that is needed clinically

Q: What is the relative sensitivity of solid and liquid phase gastric emptying studies?

A: solid phase is more sensitive; the liquid phase is always normal when the solid phase is normal

Q: When should liquid phase gastric emptying studies be performed?

A: when the patient cannot tolerate solids

Q: How long should one image to measure gastric emptying?

A: 1.5–3 hr depending on the meal used

Q: Why is attenuation correction helpful in performing gastric emptying studies?

A: movement of the meal from the posterior fundus to the anterior antrum can cause an increase in counts due to attenuation effects alone

Q: How is attenuation accounted for in gastric emptying studies?

A: obtain anterior and posterior counts and take the geometric mean

Q: When does emptying of a liquid meal begin?

A: immediately

Q: How does a coexisting solid meal affect the emptying of a liquid meal?

A: it slows the emptying of the liquid meal

Q: What is the half-life of a liquid meal in the stomach?

A: about 10–20 min

Q: When does emptying of a solid meal begin?

A: after an initial lag phase

Q: What disease can cause an increased lag phase of gastric emptying?

A: diabetes and other diseases that delay gastric emptying

Q: What is the patient preparation for a gastric emptying study?

A: overnight fast

Q: How does the urea breath test work?

A: the patient is given ^{13}C or ^{14}C labeled urea orally; the presence of ^{13}C or ^{14}C labeled CO_2 in the breath indicates urea splitting bacteria in the stomach, such as *H. pylori*, the putative cause of gastric ulcers

Q: How is gastrointestinal bleeding diagnosed using scintigraphy with ^{99m}Tc-sulfur colloid?

A: a focal area of tracer accumulation is seen that increases in intensity with time and moves within the gastrointestinal tract.

Q: What are the causes of false-positive gastrointestinal bleeding scintigraphy with ^{99m}Tc-sulfur colloid?

A: ectopic spleen, renal transplant uptake, asymmetric marrow uptake

Q: What areas of the gastrointestinal tract are difficult to diagnose gastrointestinal bleeding with ^{99m}Tc-sulfur colloid?

A: splenic flexure and transverse colon due to overlap of the liver and spleen

Q: How is a gastrointestinal bleeding scintigraphy performed with ^{99m}Tc-sulfur colloid?

A: the patient is injected with 10 mCi of ^{99m}Tc-sulfur colloid; 1 sec flow images are obtained for 60 sec followed by 1–2 min dynamic images for 20 min

Q: How is a gastrointestinal bleeding scintigraphy performed with ^{99m}Tc-RBC?

A: the patient is injected with 25 mCi of ^{99m}Tc-RBCs; 1–2 min dynamic images are obtained for 60–90 min

Q: How is gastrointestinal bleeding diagnosed using scintigraphy with ^{99m}Tc-RBCs?

A: a focal area of tracer accumulation is seen that increases in intensity with time and moves within the gastrointestinal tract

Q: What is the main advantage of ^{99m}Tc-RBCs over ^{99m}Tc-sulfur colloid for the detection of gastrointestinal bleeding?

A: the bleeding does not have to be active at the time of tracer injection resulting in greater sensitivity

Q: What drug can be given to enhance the sensitivity of gastrointestinal bleeding scintigraphy for small bowel bleeding?

A: glucagon

Q: What is the significance of large bowel activity on 24hr images in gastrointestinal bleeding scintigraphy with ^{99m}Tc-RBCs?

A: it indicates gastrointestinal bleeding, but does not localize the site; the site could have been anywhere in the gastrointestinal tract with pooling in the large intestine

Q: What rate of bleeding can be detected with gastrointestinal bleeding scintigraphy?

A: as low as 0.1 ml/min

Q: What volume of blood can be detected with gastrointestinal bleeding scintigraphy?

A: as little as 3 ml

Q: What is the whole body radiation dose of gastrointestinal bleeding scintigraphy with ^{99m}Tc-sulfur colloid?

A: 0.190 rads

Q: What is the whole body radiation dose of gastrointestinal bleeding scintigraphy with ^{99m}Tc-RBCs?

A: 0.4 rads

Q: What is the critical organ and its radiation dose for gastrointestinal bleeding scintigraphy with ^{99m}Tc-sulfur colloid?

A: the spleen with 2.1 rads

Q: What is the critical organ and its radiation dose for gastrointestinal bleeding scintigraphy with ^{99m}Tc-RBCs?

A: the heart wall with 1.4 rads

Q: What is the sensitivity and specificity of gastrointestinal scintigraphy performed with ^{99m}Tc-RBCs?

A: sensitivity: 93%; specificity: 95%

Q: What are the two main advantages of ^{99m}Tc-sulfur colloid over ^{99m}Tc-RBCs for the detection of gastrointestinal bleeding?

A: fewer false positives and the test is easier to interpret

Q: What cell type in the stomach takes up ^{99m}Tc-pertechnetate?

A: the mucin-producing parietal cells

Q: What is the target organ and its radiation dose for ^{99m}Tc-pertechnetate?

A: the stomach with 1.25 rad/5 mCi

Q: What patient preparation is required for a Meckel's scan?

A: 4–6 hr of fasting and no barium studies in the past 3–4 days

Q: What drugs are used to improve the detection of ectopic gastric mucosa with a Meckel's scan?

A: cimetidine, pentagastrin, glucagon

Q: What is the sensitivity and specificity of a Meckel's scan for ectopic gastric mucosa?

A: both approximately 80%

Q: "While buying a dozen eggs, you automatically flip open the carton to see if any are broken. This reflex is called . . ."

A: a) *apres-hen-sion*
b) *ova-sight*
c) *ovum sesame*
d) *crate eggspectations*
e) *eggsightment*
f) *dieggnosis*

Q: True/false: In jaundiced patients there is enhanced renal excretion.

A: true; with poor hepatic clearance and increased tracer in the blood pool, the degree of renal excretion is increased

Q: True/false: Some hepatomas may accumulate the hepatobiliary tracer.

A: true; most hepatocellular carcinomas are cold on IDA scans but there are some well-differentiated tumors that have demonstrated IDA uptake

Q: True/false: Serum bilirubin levels have no influence on the rate of blood pool clearance of DISIDA.

A: false; due to competitive inhibition of IDA analogues, high serum bilirubin levels interfere with tracer uptake

Q: True/false: The critical organ for IDA agents is the liver.

A: false; it is the large bowel

Q: True/false: Space-occupying lesions of the liver cannot be identified on hepatobiliary imaging.

A: false; in the early or hepatic phase of the study, cold areas can be identified

Q: True/false: Imaging in biliary atresia is more effective after phenobarbital administration.

A: true; it enhances bilirubin conjugation and excretion and also accumulation and excretion of IDA analogues

Q: True/false: Boiling is one of the steps in the preparation of Tc labeled hepatobiliary agents

A: false; boiling is one of the steps in the preparation of ^{99m}Tc-sulfur colloid, a liver and spleen imaging agent

Q: True/false: >50% of the gallbladders with acute acalculous cholecystitis are visualized on hepatobiliary imaging.

A: false; hepatobiliary imaging has high sensitivity even for acalculous cholecystitis

Q: True/false: A rim of faintly increased activity of Tc-IDA agent in the liver tissue bordering the gallbladder fossa is specific for gangrenous cholecystitis.

A: false; but it increases the likelihood

Q: True/false: Delayed or absent gall-bladder filling in a patient with impaired hepatic uptake and clearance is a reliable sign of chronic or acute cholecystitis.

A: false; delayed gallbladder filling may be caused by delayed entry of tracer into the biliary system due to poor clearance

Q: True/false: Hepatic tracer uptake of Tc-IDA is impaired in acute extrahepatic obstruction.

A: false; tracer uptake is prompt as long as hepatocyte function is intact

Q: True/false: In an adult patient, nonvisualization of the bowel at one hr is diagnostic of complete extrahepatic obstruction.

A: false; severe intrahepatic cholestasis can also give rise to a similar scan appearance

Q: True/false: Biliary tract dilatation can be reliably diagnosed on Tc-IDA scintigraphy.

A: false; ultrasound is the study of choice for assessing the caliber of the biliary ducts

Q: True/false: Obstruction of the cystic duct can be diagnosed with a reliability in excess of 90% with hepatobiliary imaging.

A: true; sensitivity is 95% or better

Q: True/false: Retrograde flow of the hepatobilary agent sufficient to allow visualization of the stomach indicates the presence of bilious gastritis.

A: false; biliary-gastric reflux does not correlate with gastric pathology and is a nonspecific finding

Q: True/false: Administration of phenobarbital in patients with hyperbilirubinemia can induce cholestasis.

A: false; it has the opposite effect

Q: True/false: Poor hepatic uptake along with nonvisualization of bowel on IDA scintigraphy are the hallmarks of biliary atresia.

A: false; good hepatic uptake with no excretion to the bowel is suggestive of biliary atresia

Q: True/false: Hepatobiliary scintigraphy has a higher sensitivity than specificity for the detection of biliary atresia.

A: true; false-positive studies can occur in cholestasis and at very high bilirubin levels

Q: True/false: Renal excretion cannot be reliably distinguished from bowel activity on IDA images.

A: false; posterior images may facilitate in distinguishing renal from bowel activity

Q: True/false: Following IV administration of sincalide, contractile response of the gallbladder can be expected after approximately 60 min.

A: false; within 10 min

Q: In liver transplant patients, is hepatobiliary scintigraphy helpful in differentiating rejection and cholestasis?

A: no; both are similar scintigraphically, with prolonged tracer retention and poor tracer clearance

Q: Following liver transplantation, the most common site for biliary leak is

_____ .

A: the anastomotic site

Q: Good hepatic uptake, persistent nonvisualization of the (CBD), along with the nonvisualization of the intestine suggests _____ .

A: acute common bile duct obstruction

Q: Nonvisualization of the gallbladder on scintigrams in the presence of a normal gallbladder can occur in _____ , _____ , and _____ .

A: postprandial patient, patients fasting >24h, patients on parenteral nutrition

Q: IDA is a structural analogue of

_____ .

A: lidocaine

Q: Following liver transplantation, the most common postoperative complication detected by biliary scintigram is

_____ .

A: biliary leak

Q: True/false: A bolus injection of sincalide is preferable to infusion over 5–10 min to obtain an accurate estimate of gallbladder ejection fraction.

A: false; rapid administration of CCK may induce gallbladder spasm and therefore impede gallbladder contraction

Q: True/false: The Kasai procedure is most successful when performed before 2 months of age.

A: true; in untreated biliary atresia, progressive hepatic injury leads to cirrhosis and hence poor response to delayed intervention

Q: True/false: Prolonged tracer uptake and clearance are typical of Dubin-Johnson syndrome.

A: false; hepatic uptake is prompt, as extraction function is intact, but excretion of organic ions into the bile is impaired; therefore, delayed clearance is characteristic

Q: True/false: Choledocal cyst often remains as a persistent cold defect in the hepatobiliary scintigraphy.

A: false; although initially they may appear as cold defects, they fill in slowly and rarely remain cold throughout the study

Q: True/false: Choledocal cysts usually respond to CCK.

A: false; a choledocal cyst is just a dilatation of the extrahepatic biliary tree with no contractile elements

Q: True/false: Intervention with morphine sulphate is contraindicated in patients with delayed gallbladder visualization.

A: false; morphine causes contraction of sphincter of oddi with increased pressure in the biliary tree, thus facilitating the entrance of the radiotracer into the cystic duct, and so is a useful technique to hasten gallbladder visualization

Q: True/false: In an elderly patient the most common cause of a lower gastro-intestinal (GI) bleed is colon carcinoma.

A: false; diverticulosis is the most common cause

Q: The most reliable technique currently available to detect upper GI bleeding is _____ .

A: upper GI endoscopy

Q: True/false: Extravasated blood usually moves antegrade in the bowel lumen.

A: false, it can move both retrograde or antegrade

Q: The critical organ for the labeled RBC technique is _____ .

A: urinary bladder (for Tc-Sc, the critical organ is the liver)

Q: True/false: The tagged RBC technique is more sensitive than Tc-Sc scanning for the detection of GI bleeding.

A: true; because of the prolonged imaging time available, intermittent bleeding can be more readily detected

Q: The minimum detectable bleeding rate for a labeled RBC study is _____ .

A: 0.5ml/min (for Tc-Sc, 0.1ml/min)

Q: The preferred radionuclide technique for the detection of lower GI bleeding is

_____ .

A: labeled (*in vitro*) RBC study

Q: True/false: Most Meckel's diverticula that become symptomatic do so during the adolescent period.

A: false; most become symptomatic during early childhood

Q: True/false: Gastric mucosa is found in approximately 50% of the Meckel's diverticula.

A: false; only 15–25% contain ectopic gastric mucosa

Q: True/false: More than 50% of the bleeding Meckel's diverticula contain ectopic gastric mucosa.

A: true

Q: Possible pharmacologic interventions that might improve the detectability of ectopic gastric mucosa are administration of _____ , _____ , or _____ .

A: pentagastrin, glucagon, cimetidine

Q: True/false: A patient with inferior vena cava (IVC) obstruction injected in the antecubital fossa with ^{99m}Tc-Sc intravenously will demonstrate a hot quadrate lobe.

A: false; (SVC) obstruction can result in a hot quadrate lobe

Q: True/false: Routine SPECT imaging in liver-spleen scans yield higher sensitivity and specificity.

A: false; sensitivity may be increased but specificity suffers

Q: True/false: Albumin colloid is an alternative liver and spleen imaging agent.

A: true

Q: Delayed biliary-to-bowel transit on a HIDA scan may be indicative of:
a. opiate effect
b. chronic cholecystitis
c. other inflammatory conditions in abdomen
d. any of the above

A: d

Q: Total retention of IDA in the hepatic parenchyma over a 4-hr time period in an acutely ill patient is reflective of:
a. cystic duct obstruction
b. hepatic parenchymal disease
c. partial common duct obstruction
d. complete common duct obstruction

A: d

Match the following three pharmacologic interventions with their clinical usages in HIDA scintigraphy:
a. bilary atresia
b. given 20–30 min after ^{99m}Tc-IDA to speed the completion of study for suspected acute cholecystitis
c. biliary dyskinesis

Q: phenobarbital

A: a

Q: morphine

A: b

Q: sincalide

A: c

Q: True/false: The iminodiacetic acid group of hepatobiliary radiopharmaceuticals are similar to bilirubin in that they are conjugated in the liver.

A: false

Q: Which of the following disorders is usually associated with an enhanced blood pool on a labeled RBC study of the liver?
a. hemangioma
b. hepatoma
c. metastatic disease
d. focal nodular hyperplasia
e. all of the above

A: a

Q: The term *colloid shift* is generally associated with:
a. metastatic disease
b. hepatoma
c. cirrhosis
d. all of the above
e. none of the above

A: c

Q: Space-occupying lesions of the liver that generally concentrate ^{67}Ga citrate include:
a. lymphoma
b. hepatoma
c. abscess
d. all of the above
e. none of the above

A: d

Q: True/false: *In vitro* labeling of RBCs is more effective than the modified *in vivtro* method.

A: true

Q: ^{99m}Tc-pertechnetate abdominal imaging may be used to detect:
a. Barrett's esophagitis
b. Meckel's diverticulum
c. retained gastric antrum
d. all of the above

A: d

Q: All of the following have been proposed as pharmacologic interventions to enhance Meckel's diverticulum imaging except:
a. cholestryramine
b. pentagastin
c. glucagon
d. cimetidine

A: a

Q: The normal half-time of gastric emptying of a labeled solid meal is:
a. 30–45 min
b. 45–60 min
c. 75–90 min
d. 90–120 min

A: c

Q: Significantly prolonged esophageal transit often is associated with:
a. scleroderma
b. achalasia
c. diabetes mellitus
d. a and b
e. all of the above

A: d

Q: The current radiopharmaceutical of choice for confirming patency of Le Veen shunts (after intraperitoneal installation) is:
a. ^{99m}Tc-MAG 3
b. ^{111}In-DTPA
c. ^{99m}Tc-sulfur colloid
d. ^{99m}Tc-MAA

A: d

Q: True/false: Warthin's tumors of the parotid gland generally show avid uptake of ^{99m}Tc-pertechnetate.

A: true

Q: What class of radiopharmaceuticals is used for cholescintigraphy?

A: ^{99m}Tc-iminodiacetic acid analogs (IDA)

Q: What are the two agents approved by the FDA for cholescintigraphy?

A: ^{99m}Tc-disofenin and ^{99m}Tc-mebrofenin

Q: Why is ^{99m}Tc-IDA called bifunctional chelates?

A: one end of the molecule is polar and anionic and binds to ^{99m}Tc; the other end of the molecule is lipophilic and determines the molecule's biologic function

Q: How many IDA molecules does it take to chelate one ^{99m}Tc molecule?

A: two

Q: What physiologic molecule does ^{99m}Tc-IDA most closely mimic?

A: bilirubin

Q: Why is ^{99m}Tc-IDA not excreted by the kidneys?

A: it is protein bound in the circulation

Q: What is the main difference between the metabolism of ^{99m}Tc-IDA and bilirubin?

A: ^{99m}Tc-IDA is not conjugated

Q: What factors determine the differential flow of excreted ^{99m}Tc-IDA into the gall bladder versus the duodenum?

A: the patency of the cystic ducts, the tone of the sphincter of oddi, and intraluminal pressures

Q: What level of bilirubin is required to interfere with the quality of a ^{99m}Tc-mebrofenin or ^{99m}Tc-disofenin scan?

A: over 20–30 mg/dl

Q: What is the alternate route of excretion of ^{99m}Tc-IDA with severe hepatocellular function?

A: renal

Q: What percentage of a dose of ^{99m}Tc-mebrofenin is taken up by the liver?

A: 98%

Q: What percentage of a dose of ^{99m}Tc-disofenin is taken up by the liver?

A: 98%

Q: What is the biologic half-life of ^{99m}Tc-mebrofenin in the blood?

A: 17 min

Q: What is the biologic half-life of ^{99m}Tc-disofenin in the blood?

A: 19 min

Q: What percentage of a dose of ^{99m}Tc-mebrofenin is excreted by the kidney?

A: <1%

Q: What percentage of a dose of ^{99m}Tc-disofenin is excreted by the kidney?

A: <9%

Q: What is the critical organ for ^{99m}Tc-mebrofenin and ^{99m}Tc-disofenin and what is its radiation dose?

A: the liver with 1.9 Rads/5 mCi

Q: How long should a patient be fasting before cholescintigraphy, and why?

A: 4 hours, to wait for postprandial (CCK) levels to normalize

Q: What is the maximum time that a patient should be fasting before cholescintigraphy, and why?

A: 24 hrs; after 24 hrs, the gallbladder may be too tensely filled with bile to take up tracer

Q: How should patients with a prolonged fasting state be prepared before cholescintigraphy?

A: injection of CCK or sincalide

Q: What is the cause of visualization of the liver at the same time as the liver and the spleen on the blood flow phase of cholescintigraphy?

A: arterialization of the flow to the liver, which may be seen in cirrhosis or involvement of the liver by tumor

Q: What is the routine adult dose of ^{99m}Tc-disofenin or ^{99m}Tc-mebrofenin?

A: 5.0 mCi

Q: What is the minimum dose of ^{99m}Tc-disofenin or ^{99m}Tc-mebrofenin for a child?

A: 1 mCi

Q: What type of collimator should be used for cholescintigraphy?

A: low-energy, all-purpose parallel hole

Q: What type of computer acquisition should be used for cholescintigraphy?

A: 1 min dynamic images for 60 min with an optional flow study (1 sec images for 60 sec)

Q: How is hepatic clearance of the tracer assessed?

A: compare the 5 min image of liver uptake to the 1 min blood pool image and look for clearing of the heart's blood pool by 5 min

Q: In a normal person, when is biliary excretion seen on cholescintigraphy?

A: at about 10 min

Q: How accurate is cholescintigraphy for anatomically sizing ducts?

A: it is not accurate and should not be used for this purpose

Q: In a normal fasting person, what percentage of excreted bile enters the gallbladder?

A: one-third

Q: When is the normal gallbladder usually seen on cholescintigraphy?

A: on average, at about 20 min and always within 60 min

Q: In a normal person, when is the bowel activity seen on cholescintigraphy?

A: 30 min; however, 10–20% of normal patients will have delayed biliary-to-bowel transit beyond 60 min

Q: How can one distinguish physiologically delayed biliary-to-bowel transit time from partial common bile duct obstruction on cholescintigraphy?

A: obtain delayed images or administer sincalide

Q: How should sincalide be administered?

A: over several min intravenously

Q: How long do you need to wait between administration of sincalide and dosing for cholescintigraphy?

A: at least 30 min

Q: How does prior sincalide administration affect the biliary-to-bowel transit time on cholescintigraphy?

A: sincalide delays biliary-to-bowel transit time

Q: When performing cholescintigraphy, why should sincalide not be given after morphine?

A: morphine will counteract the effects of sincalide

Q: How can one distinguish acute from chronic cholecystitis as a cause of nonvisualization of the gallbladder at 1 hr on cholescintigraphy?

A: obtain delayed images and perform morphine augmentation

Q: What two scintigraphic findings on cholescintigraphy increase the likelihood that nonvisualization of the gallbladder is caused by acute cholecystitis?

A: hyperemia in the gallbladder fossa on early phase images or a rim sign on later images

Q: What percentage of patients with acute cholecystitis have a rim sign on cholescintigraphy?

A: 25%

Q: What is the prognostic implication of a rim sign on cholescintigraphy?

A: it is associated with gallbladder gangrene and perforation

Q: How does morphine-augmented cholescintigraphy work?

A: morphine increases the tone of the sphincter of oddi, thereby raising common bile duct pressure, and facilitating gallbladder filling, if the cystic duct is patent

Q: How does one perform morphine-augmented cholescintigraphy?

A: if the gallbladder does not fill by 60 min on routine cholescintigraphy, give 0.04 mg/kg of morphine IV; if the gallbladder does not fill within an additional 30 min, the patient has cystic duct obstruction

Q: What is the major cause of a false-negative scan for acute cholecystitis on cholescintigraphy?

A: acute acalculous cholecystitis

Q: How does one perform a gallbladder ejection fraction?

A: administer sincalide 0.02 μg/kg intravenously over several min; a normal gallbladder ejection fraction is greater than 35%

Q: What patient preparation is required before cholescintigraphy for the diagnosis of congenital biliary atresia?

A: phenobarbital 5 mg/kg for 5 days

Q: What are the specific scintigraphic findings of partial common bile duct obstruction on cholescintigraphy?

A: common bile duct showing segmental narrowing, abrupt or gradual cutoff, filling defects, or activity that does not decrease on delayed images

Q: How does one identify choledochal cyst on cholescintigraphy?

A: the cyst fills with tracer, although delayed images may be required to document filling

Q: Why do large cavernous hemangioma have inhomogeneous uptake on a ^{99m}Tc-RBC scan?

A: because of thromboses within the hemangioma

Q: What is the positive predictive value of a positive ^{99m}Tc-RBC scan for cavernous hemangioma?

A: >99%

Q: What is the sensitivity of planar and SPECT imaging for detection of cavernous hemangioma with ^{99m}Tc-RBCs?

A: planar: 60–70%; SPECT: 85–90%

Q: How small a hemangioma can be seen with planar and SPECT ^{99m}Tc-RBC imaging?

A: planar: 3 cm; SPECT: 1.5 cm

Q: What two tracers are available for liver–spleen scanning?

A: ^{99m}Tc-sulfur colloid and ^{99m}Tc-albumin colloid

Q: What is the blood clearance half-life of ^{99m}Tc-sulfur colloid?

A: 2–3 min

Q: What fractions of an intravenous dose of ^{99m}Tc-sulfur colloid localize in the liver, spleen, and bone marrow?

A: liver: 85%; spleen: 10%; bone marrow: 5%

Q: What cells in the liver take up ^{99m}Tc-sulfur colloid?

A: the Kupffer cells

Q: How does an increased number of small particles affect the organ distribution of colloids?

A: smaller particle sizes tend to localize in the marrow

Q: How does an increased number of large particles affect the organ distribution of colloids?

A: larger particle sizes tend to localize in the liver

Q: What is a colloid shift and its causes?

A: decreased uptake of colloid by the liver and increased uptake by the spleen caused by liver dysfunction or a shift in blood flow (e.g. portal hypertension)

Q: What is the main difference in the preparation of ^{99m}Tc-sulfur colloid and ^{99m}Tc-albumin colloid?

A: ^{99m}Tc-sulfur colloid requires heating, while ^{99m}Tc-albumin colloid does not

Q: What is the contraindication to ^{99m}Tc-albumin colloid?

A: hypersensitivity to albumin-containing products

Q: What is the typical appearance of a benign lesion of the liver on ^{99m}Tc-sulfur colloid liver–spleen scanning?

A: cold lesion

Q: What is the typical appearance of a malignant lesion of the liver on ^{99m}Tc-sulfur colloid liver–spleen scanning?

A: cold lesion

Q: How does radiation therapy affect liver uptake of ^{99m}Tc-sulfur colloid?

A: it causes rectangular-shaped defects

Q: What is the typical cause of a hot quadrate lobe of the liver on ^{99m}Tc-sulfur colloid imaging?

A: superior vena cava obstruction

Q: What is the typical cause of a hot caudate lobe of the liver on ^{99m}Tc-sulfur colloid imaging?

A: Budd-Chiari syndrome (hepatic vein thrombosis)

Q: What liver tumor can show increased uptake of ^{99m}Tc-sulfur colloid?

A: focal nodular hyperplasia

Q: What size of liver lesions can be reliably detected on planar images of a ^{99m}Tc-sulfur colloid liver–spleen scan?

A: 2–3 cm

Q: What size of liver lesions can be reliably detected on SPECT images of a ^{99m}Tc-sulfur colloid liver–spleen scan?

A: 1.5–2.0 cm

Q: What agent can be used to specifically image the spleen with minimal liver uptake?

A: ^{99m}Tc-heat-damaged RBCs

9 Genitourinary

Q: Scintigraphic renal agents that are excreted by the kidney and measure effective renal plasma flow (ERPF) include _____ .

A: ^{99m}Tc-MAG$_3$, ^{123}I-orthoiodohippuran, and ^{131}I-orthoiodohippuran

Q: The percentage of ^{131}I-OIH that is filtered by the kidneys is _____ .

A: 20%

Q: To perform a flow study with a ^{99m}Tc-labeled radiopharmaceutical, one must inject at least _____ .

A: 10–15 mCi as a bolus with rapid sequence scintiphotos

Q: Which agent should one choose if flow images and ERPF are to be evaluated?

A: ^{99m}Tc-MAG$_3$

Q: The scintigraphic renal imaging agent that is primarily filtered and may be used to determine the glomerular filtration rate is _____ .

A: ^{99m}Tc-DTPA

Q: Scintigraphic renal agents that are used to assess the appearance of the renal parenchyma include _____ .

A: ^{99m}Tc-dimercaptosuccinic acid (DMSA) and ^{99m}Tc-glucoheptonate (GHA)

Q: The scintigraphic renal cortical imaging agent that also demonstrates the collecting system on early images is _____ .

A: ^{99m}Tc-GHA

Q: Compared to ^{99m}Tc-GHA, the renal transit time of ^{99m}Tc-DMSA is _____ .

A: longer

Q: The percentage of ^{99m}Tc-GHA retained by the kidneys is approximately _____ .

A: 15%

Q: The scintigraphic renal cortical imaging agent that reaches the highest concentration in the cortex (42% of the injected dose) is _____ .

A: ^{99m}Tc-DMSA

Q: Of the most commonly used renal imaging agents, the one that gives the highest radiation dose to the kidneys per mCi is _____ .

A: ^{99m}Tc-DMSA

Q: If a flow study and cortical imaging are to be performed, one should choose _____ .

A: ^{99m}Tc-GHA, because of the lower cortical radiation dose

Q: What scintigraphic renal imaging agent is structurally related to para-aminohippurate?

A: ^{131}I or ^{123}I-orthoiodohippuran (OIH)

Q: A radiopharmaceutical that is usually taken up by a suspected renal abscess is _____ .

A: ^{67}Ga-citrate

Q: The kidneys are normally not well visualized on a ^{67}Ga-citrate scan after _____ .

A: 24 hr

Q: The kidneys receive approximately _____ percent of cardiac output.

A: 25

Q: The normal adult glomerular filtration rate is _____ .

A: 125 ml/min

Q: The normal adult renal blood flow is _____ .

A: 1250 ml/min

Q: The normal adult renal plasma flow is _____ .

A: 700 ml/min

Q: The renal blood vessel that carries blood directly away from the glomerulus is called the _____ .

A: efferent arteriole

Q: Regarding the radiorenogram curve, which portion of the curve is most affected by dehydration?

A: transit

Q: Which portion of the renogram curve is most affected by acute obstruction?

A: excretion

Q: When determining the percent function, which portion of the radiorenogram curve is utilized?

A: uptake

Q: What nonradioactive pharmaceutical is often administered to distinguish an obstructed dilated collection system from a nonobstructed dilated collection system during radiorenography?

A: furosemide (lasix)

Q: In a nonobstructed kidney, the washout half-time on a postlasix (furosamide) renogram is less than _____ minutes.

A: 10

Q: In an obstructed kidney, the washout half-time on a postlasix (furosamide) renogram is generally greater than _____ minutes.

A: 20

Q: When processing the renogram data, the background regions of interest are usually placed _____ .

A: inferolaterally

Q: In children, the most common site of renal obstruction is at the _____ .

A: ureteropelvic junction

Q: The site of renal obstruction in adults is most common at the _____ .

A: uretero-vesicular junction

Q: Is an agent more likely to be filtered or secreted if it is highly protein bound?

A: secreted

Q: What substance traditionally has been used to determine the glomerular filtration rate (GFR) by non-nuclear medicine techniques?

A: inulin

Q: The simplest way to reduce the radiation exposure to the bladder after a radionuclide renal study is by _____ .

A: having the patient void

Q: By definition, the filtration fraction is the ratio of _____ .

A: GFR to ERPF, i.e., FF = GFR/ERPF

Q: On a normal renal flow study, the kidneys should be visualized _____ .

A: at the same time as the aorta and iliac vessels

Q: During the course of a renal radionuclide study, a rising background curve can be seen most commonly when _____ .

A: the dose has infiltrated

Q: Two main pathologic processes that cause renal artery stenosis are _____ .

A: fibromuscular dysplasia and atherosclerotic disease

Q: The mechanism of action of captopril is _____ .

A: blockade of the conversion of angiotensin I to angiotensin II

Q: Regarding captopril renography of a patient with renal artery stenosis, what parameter of renal function is most affected on the postcaptopril study, and in what way?

A: the GFR is reduced

Q: The dose of captopril usually administered for a captopril renogram is _____ .

A: 25mg or 50 mg (po)

Q: At what time intervals should images be obtained for renal flow studies?

A: rapid sequence scintigrams at 2–5 sec intervals for 1 min.

Q: On a renal flow study, the liver is visualized after the kidneys because _____ .

A: the majority of blood supply to the liver is via the hepatic portal system, not arterial

Q: The typical adult dose for a ^{99m}Tc-MAG$_3$ renogram without a flow study is _____ .

A: 2–4 mCi IV

Q: What is the scintigraphic appearance of a lymphocele?

A: photopenic area adjacent to the transplanted kidney

Q: What is thought to be the cause of lymphocele formation?

A: ligation or disruption of regional lymphatic vessels

Q: The scintigraphic appearance of a hypertrophied column of Bertin is _____ .

A: an area of tissue with normal function, similar to the surrounding renal parenchyma

Q: In kidneys with a duplicated collection system, obstruction more commonly occurs in _____ .

A: the upper collecting system

Q: The most common abnormality of fusion involving the kidneys is _____ .

A: horseshoe kidney

Q: At what anatomic location do dromedary humps occur?

A: lateral margin, left kidney

Q: The _____ pole of the kidney may appear more photopenic because it is located further from the camera when imaging posteriorly.

A: lower

Q: In a normal patient, using 3-min. scintirenograms, the renal pelves and collection systems should be visualized initially on which image?

A: the second image (3–6 min)

Q: The renal process that requires no expenditure of metabolic energy is _____ .

A: glomerular filtration

Q: Patient preparation performed for a nuclear medicine renal study should include _____ .

A: hydration and emptying of the bladder

Q: If a patient 1 month post-transplant who has received antirejection medications, begins to have delayed excretion with relatively perserved perfusion, one should consider _____ .

A: cyclosporin toxicity

Q: When performing a renogram on a post-transplant patient, the gamma camera is typically placed _____ .

A: anteriorly over the pelvic transplant site

Q: The typical scintigraphic appearance of a renal cyst is _____ .

A: a round photopenic area within normal renal parenchyma

Q: On a renal parenchymal study, a wedge-shaped defect extending to the periphery of an involved kidney may represent _____ .

A: an infarct or pyelonephritis

Q: Regarding early post-transplant renograms, a pattern of normal uptake and delayed, but not absent, excretion is most consistent with what diagnosis?

A: acute tubular necrosis

Q: The etiology of hyperacute renal transplant rejection is _____ .

A: undetected preformed antibodies in the host

Q: The time frame for hyperacute renal transplant rejection is _____ .

A: within 24 hrs of transplant

Q: The type of renal transplant rejection that occurs several days to several weeks post-transplantation is termed _____ .

A: acute rejection

Q: The scintigraphic findings consistent with renal transplant rejection are _____ .

A: delayed flow and poor excretion worsening over time

Q: Is the perfusion to a transplanted kidney worse with ATN or with rejection?

A: rejection

Q: The type of renal transplant rejection that is predominantly mediated by cellular immune mechanisms is _____ .

A: chronic rejection

Q: Where are most sites of urine extravasation found in post-transplant patients?

A: at the ureto-vesical anastomosis

Q: What diagnosis should be considered in a renal transplant patient when there is an area of photopenia near the kidney that progressively demonstrates increased uptake with time?

A: urinoma (bladder must first be excluded)

Q: Approximately _____ % of adults with polycystic liver disease have polycystic kidneys.

A: 50

Q: _____ % of medullary sponge kidney disease is bilateral.

A: 75

Q: Which disease is more life-threatening, infantile polycystic renal disease or medullary sponge kidney disease?

A: infantile polycystic disease is typically bilateral and fatal

Q: At what vertebral levels are the kidneys usually located?

A: upper poles at T11 and lower poles near L3

Q: Which kidney is more frequently ptotic?

A: the right kidney

Q: Which kidney is more frequently ectopic?

A: the left kidney

Q: The renal tumor common in patients with tuberous sclerosis is
_____ .

A: hamartoma (angiomyolipoma)

Q: Although nonspecific, the typical scintigraphic appearance of Wilm's tumor is _____ .

A: decreased uptake with variable vascular pattern

Q: What is the most common metastatic tumor to the kidneys?

A: lymphoma

Q: On a renogram where sharp, straight margins adjacent to decreased uptake of the radiotracer are present, one should consider what diagnosis?

A: radiation nephritis

Q: What are the two main methods to perform radionuclide cystography?

A: direct and indirect cystography

Q: Grade 1 reflux signifies
_____ .

A: urinary reflux into the ureter only

Q: Grade _____ reflux occurs when there is reflux into a dilated ureter and renal pelvis.

A: 3

Q: What radiopharmaceuticals are used to perform direct cystography?

A: ^{99m}Tc-pertechnetate or ^{99m}Tc-sulfur colloid

Q: Which is more sensitive for detecting reflux, a radionuclide cystogram or a contrast cystogram (VCUG)?

A: radionuclide cystogram

Q: Which radionuclide cystographic technique allows one to also evaluate renal function?

A: the indirect radionuclide cystogram

Q: Approximately what percentage of patients demonstrate reflux only during filling?

A: 20%

Q: What is the main disadvantage of the direct radionuclide cystogram technique?

A: it requires bladder catheterization

Q: A radionuclide cystogram that shows a "Mickey Mouse ears" pattern suggests what?

A: bilateral vesico-ureteral reflux

Q: What position is a young child placed in when performing a radionuclide cystogram?

A: lying with the camera positioned posteriorly

Q: In general, what are the three phases of a direct radionuclide cystogram?

A: filling, voiding, and postvoiding images

Q: What is the average bladder capacity of a child?

A: (age +2) $\times$ 30 ml

Q: Residual urine volume can be determined after what radionuclide techniques?

A: direct or indirect cystography and after a renal scan

Q: The anatomic anomaly often associated with testicular torsion is _____ .

A: "bell clapper" anomaly

Q: The radiopharmaceutical generally used for testicular scanning is _____ .

A: ^{99m}Tc-pertechnetate

Q: The major phases of a radionuclide testicular study are _____ .

A: flow images, static scrotal images, and delayed pinhole images

Q: In addition to performing pinhole images, what maneuver is typically performed to improve accuracy and clarify anatomy?

A: placement of lead markers

Q: During the flow study, the _____ sign can be occasionally visualized and has a high specificity for testicular torsion.

A: "nubbin"

Q: On static delayed images testicular torsion appears as _____ .

A: a photopenic defect surrounded by normal scrotal activity

Q: A photopenic defect in the region of the testis surrounded by hyperemia of the scrotum is suggestive of (but not specific for) _____ .

A: late torsion

Q: A common disorder that may present with testicular pain but is treated conservatively is _____ .

A: epididymitis or epididymo-orchitis

Q: The appearance of epidydmitis/orchitis on scrotal scintigraphy is _____ .

A: hyperemia of the involved epidydimus/testicle, often with increased flow seen on the dynamic images as well

Match the following six statements with the most appropriate radiopharmaceutical:
a. ^{99m}Tc-DTPA
b. ^{99m}Tc-glucoheptonate
c. ^{99m}Tc-DMSA
d. ^{99m}Tc-MAG-3
e. ^{131}I-orthoiodohippurate

Q: handled by GFR (20%) and tubular secretion (80%)

A: e

Q: clearance best approximates the normal ERPF of 600 ml/min

A: e

Q: actively secreted by tubules with no significant filtration

A: d

Q: more than 40% of the administered dose binds to the tubules

A: c

Q: normal ERPF is between 400 and 500 ml/min

A: d

Q: associated with lowest radiation dose to the kidney per administered mCi

A: d

Q: True/false: Captopril acts by blocking the production of angiotensin I.

A: false

Q: During captopril scintigraphy, a renovascular etiology for hypertension will most often cause delay in:
a. perfusion to the affected kidney
b. cortical uptake in the affected kidney
c. transit from cortex to collecting system in affected kidney
d. excretion from the affected kidney

A: c

Q: Following intravenous furosemide, the normal half-time of disappearance of collecting system activity in a nonobstructed kidney should not exceed:
a. 1–3 min
b. 8–12 min
c. 15–20 min
d. less than 30 min

A: b

Q: True/false: Renal cell carcinomas generally show increased concentration of glucoheptonate compared to normal surrounding renal parenchyma.

A: false

Q: In renal transplant evaluation, ATN typically is associated with:
a. poor perfusion, slow but good uptake, slow, progressive excretion
b. poor perfusion, poor uptake, slow progressive excretion
c. good perfusion, slow but good uptake, little or no excretion
d. good perfusion, poor uptake, little or no excretion

A: d

Q: In renal transplant evaluation, chronic rejection typically is associated with:
a. poor perfusion, slow but good uptake, slow, progressive excretion
b. poor perfusion, poor uptake, slow progressive excretion
c. good perfusion, slow but good uptake, little or no excretion
d. good perfusion, poor uptake, little or no excretion

A: b

Q: Quantitative or semiquantitative determination of individual renal function can be achieved with:
a. ^{99m}Tc-MAG-3
b. ^{99m}Tc-DTPA
c. ^{99m}Tc-DMSA
d. ^{131}I-hippuran
e. all of the above

A: e

Q: True/false: Static "morphologic" images with glucoheptonate are not as sensitive as urography or sonography in detecting pyelonephritis.

A: false

Q: In scrotal imaging, a "photon-deficient" area surrounded by a rim of increased activity is typical of:
a. hydrocoele
b. seminoma
c. late testicular torsion
d. torsion of the appendix testes
e. all of the above

A: c

Q: True/false: In some patients, vesico-ureteral (V-U) reflux occurs only during bladder filling and not during voiding.

A: true

Q: True/false: When studying a patient for V-U reflux, the indirect method of radionuclide cystography effectively evaluates all phases of bladder filling and emptying.

A: false

10 Infection, Inflammation, and Tumor

Q: What element does ^{67}Ga most closely mimic in terms of biologic behavior?

A: iron (Fe-III)

Q: How is ^{67}Ga produced?

A: by cyclotron bombardment of ^{68}Zn

Q: How does ^{67}Ga decay?

A: electron capture

Q: What is the half-life of ^{67}Ga?

A: 78 hr

Q: What are energies of the principle photons of ^{67}Ga decay?

A: 93, 185, 300, and 394 keV

Q: What photopeaks of ^{67}Ga are most commonly used for imaging?

A: 93 and 185keV

Q: To what serum protein does ^{67}Ga bind after injection?

A: transferrin

Q: Why does gallium not become incorporated into heme and other similar iron-containing compounds?

A: incorporation of iron into heme requires the reduction of Fe from the +3 to the +2 oxidation state; gallium cannot be reduced by the body to a 2+ state

Q: What percentage of a dose of ^{67}Ga is excreted by the kidneys in the first 24 hr after injection?

A: 15–25%

Q: What is the biologic half-life of ^{67}Ga excretion beyond 24 hr after injection?

A: 25 days

Q: What is the major route of ^{67}Ga excretion beyond 24 hr after injection?

A: the gastrointestinal tract

Q: How does iron overload affect ^{67}Ga biodistribution?

A: it saturates transferrin and causes less liver uptake and more renal excretion and bone uptake

Q: What mechanisms cause ^{67}Ga uptake by tumors?

A: increased vascular permeability of tumors, transferrin receptors on tumors, and increased concentration of iron-binding proteins in tumors

Q: How does ^{67}Ga uptake differ between viable and necrotic tumor?

A: ^{67}Ga is only taken up by viable tumor and will not be taken up by necrotic tumor

Q: How does the dose of ^{67}Ga used for tumor detection generally differ from the dose used for inflammation detection?

A: a larger dose is given for tumor detection

Q: What is the usual dose of ^{67}Ga for tumor detection?

A: 10 mCi

Q: What is the critical organ for ^{67}Ga dosimetry, and what is its radiation-absorbed dose?

A: the large intestine, with a dose of 9 rads/10 mCi

Q: Why is there great variation in the medical literature regarding the utility of ^{67}Ga for tumor detection?

A: most of it was published before 1985 using lower doses and no SPECT

Q: How many photopeaks of ^{67}Ga should be detected for tumor detection?

A: at least two and preferably three

Q: How many counts should be obtained for planar ^{67}Ga images for tumor detection?

A: at least 500K counts for routine whole body images and at least 1000K counts for evaluation of areas of previous disease

Q: When should images be obtained with ^{67}Ga for tumor detection?

A: at about 2–3 days and 7–10 days after injection

Q: What is the advantage of performing sequential SPECT examinations with ^{67}Ga imaging for tumor detection?

A: sequential SPECT examinations help differentiate pathologic abdominal uptake from physiologic bowel localization

Q: How much time should elapse between treatment with chemotherapy and ^{67}Ga imaging to assess tumor response?

A: 3–6 weeks

Q: How can inflammation and tumor be differentiated when there is ^{67}Ga uptake in hilar lymph nodes?

A: ^{201}Tl imaging will show uptake in tumor but not in inflammation

Q: How does normal spleen uptake of ^{67}Ga compare to normal liver uptake?

A: spleen uptake is less than the liver

Q: What organs normally take up ^{67}Ga?

A: liver, spleen, bone marrow, salivary glands, lacrimal glands, nasal mucosa, external genitalia, female breast

Q: What physiologic condition results in markedly increased female breast uptake?

A: lactation

Q: What condition can cause increased salivary gland uptake of ^{67}Ga unrelated to tumor or infection?

A: head/neck radiation therapy

Q: What organ in the chest may show physiologic uptake of ^{67}Ga in children?

A: thymus

Q: For how long is kidney uptake normal on a ^{67}Ga scan?

A: 24 hr

Q: What are the causes of faint liver uptake on ⁶⁷Ga imaging?

A: competition for uptake by tumor, liver dysfunction, recent administration of chemotherapy (vincristine), iron overload, and increased renal clearance

Q: What are the causes of increased kidney uptake on ⁶⁷Ga imaging that are unrelated to infection or tumor?

A: hepatic or renal failure, recent chemotherapy (vincristine and Cytoxan), recent transfusion

Q: For how long can uninfected surgical wounds have increased uptake after ⁶⁷Ga?

A: 1–2 weeks

Q: How does lymphangiography affect ⁶⁷Ga uptake?

A: it can cause diffusely increased lung uptake

Q: What procedure increases the sensitivity of ⁶⁷Ga to the detection of affected axillary lymph nodes?

A: imaging patients with their arms raised

Q: Why are large tumor deposits sometimes missed on ⁶⁷Ga imaging?

A: larger tumors commonly undergo necrosis and no longer take up ⁶⁷Ga

Q: What procedure improves the detection of tumor in the liver or spleen by ⁶⁷Ga?

A: comparison with a sulfur colloid study to look for areas of decreased uptake on colloid scan that fill in with ⁶⁷Ga

Q: What is the complication of using vigorous enemas and bowel preparations for ⁶⁷Ga imaging?

A: they can cause bowel inflammation that takes up ⁶⁷Ga

Q: What is the sensitivity of ⁶⁷Ga for detecting Hodgkin's lymphoma?

A: about 90%

Q: What histologic types of Hodgkin's lymphoma have the highest and lowest sensitivities for detection by ⁶⁷Ga?

A: highest: nodular sclerosing, mixed cellularity, and lymphocyte depleted; lowest: lymphocyte predominant

Q: What is the sensitivity of ⁶⁷Ga imaging for detecting high-grade non-Hodgkin's lymphomas?

A: about 85–90%

Q: How does the sensitivity of ⁶⁷Ga to low- and intermediate-grade non-Hodgkin's lymphomas compare to the higher-grade non-Hodgkin's lymphomas?

A: it is less

Q: What is the main use of ⁶⁷Ga imaging in lymphoma?

A: to determine tumor viability after chemotherapy

Q: How is ⁶⁷Ga imaging used to detect tumor viability?

A: a pretherapy scan is needed to confirm gallium uptake; post-therapy uptake indicates persistent viable tumor

Q: How is ⁶⁷Ga useful in diagnosing hepatomas?

A: it can be used to distinguish hepatomas from regeneration nodules

Q: What percentage of hepatomas are gallium avid?

A: 90%

Q: What percentage of hepatomas show uptake greater than the normal liver?

A: 50%

Q: How is ^{67}Ga useful in the management of lung cancer?

A: ^{67}Ga scans can show mediastinal lymph nodes and distant metastases whose presence precludes surgical resection

Q: What is the sensitivity of ^{67}Ga imaging for lung cancer?

A: 85–90%

Q: What is the sensitivity of ^{67}Ga imaging for colon cancer?

A: 25%

Q: What is the sensitivity of ^{67}Ga imaging for pancreatic cancer?

A: 15%

Q: What is the sensitivity of ^{67}Ga imaging for soft tissue sarcomas?

A: 90–95%

Q: What element does ^{201}Tl mimic in the body?

A: potassium

Q: How does ^{201}Tl decay?

A: electron capture

Q: What are the photopeaks of ^{201}Tl?

A: a cluster of X rays from 69–83 keV and gamma rays at 135 and 167 keV

Q: What percentage of a dose of ^{201}Tl goes to the heart?

A: 3–5%

Q: What is the critical organ for intravenous ^{201}Tl chloride, and what is the radiation-absorbed dose?

A: the kidneys, with a dose of 3.6 rad/mCi

Q: When should imaging begin after ^{201}Tl injection for tumor detection?

A: 10–30 min

Q: Does ^{201}Tl imaging correlate with the histologic grade of primary brain glial tumors?

A: yes, the higher the uptake, the higher the tumor grade

Q: Does ^{201}Tl imaging differentiate brain tumor recurrence from radiation necrosis?

A: yes, tumor recurrence shows uptake, while radiation necrosis shows no uptake

Q: How is ^{201}Tl imaging useful for evaluating intracranial lesions in patients with AIDS?

A: uptake in the brain indicates lymphoma or other malignancy; no uptake suggests an infectious cause

Q: How is ^{201}Tl imaging useful in the management of primary bone tumors?

A: it accurately detects the extent of involvement and predicts and assesses the response to chemotherapy

Q: What is the advantage of ^{201}Tl imaging over ^{131}I imaging for detecting thyroid cancer?

A: ^{201}Tl imaging does not require withdrawal of thyroid hormone treatment

Q: What is the main advantage of ^{131}I imaging over ^{201}Tl imaging for the detection of thyroid cancer?

A: ^{131}I imaging predicts the potential usefulness of ^{131}I therapy

Q: In a patient with a history of thyroid cancer and a negative I-131 scan, when is a ^{201}Tl scan indicated?

A: when the serum thyroglobulin level is elevated

Q: How is ^{201}Tl imaging useful in the evaluation of Kaposi's sarcoma?

A: Kaposi's sarcoma is usually negative on gallium imaging, but is positive on thallium imaging

Q: What are two advantages of using antibody fragments over the whole antibodies for immunoscintigraphy?

A: more rapid clearance and less antigenicity

Q: What is the tracer of choice to image parathyroid adenomas?

A: ^{99m}Tc-sestamibi

Q: What imaging agent is available to image adrenal medullary tumors?

A: ^{131}I metaiodobenzylguanidine (MIBG)

Q: What is the name of a technetium labelled radioimmunoscintigraphic agent for colon cancer?

A: CEAscan

Q: What is the name of a ^{111}Indium labelled monoclonal antibody for imaging ovarian and colorectal carcinomas?

A: OncoScint

Q: What imaging agent is available to image adrenal cortical tumors:

A: ^{131}NP-59 (6-beta-iodomethyl-19-norcholesterol

Q: In what region of the body is OncoScint scanning more sensitive than CT for recurrent ovarian cancer?

A: in the abdomen outside the liver

Q: When are patients imaged after injection with OncoScint?

A: at 24–48 hr and at 72–120 hr after injection

Q: What is the critical organ and its radiation-absorbed dose for OncoScint?

A: liver, 15 Rad / 5 mCi

Q: What percentage of patients develop HAMA after injection with OncoScint?

A: 40%

Q: In what percentage of patients who develop HAMA do the antibodies eventually go away?

A: 50%

Q: How can HAMA interfere with diagnostic tests?

A: they can cause false-positive assays of carcinoembryonic antigen (CEA) and ^{125}Ca

Q: What are the humanized antibodies for radioimmunoscintigraphy?

A: antibodies in which the variable region comes from mouse DNA and the fixed region comes from human DNA

Q: What are the main organs that can be seen normally after injection of OncoScint?

A: liver, spleen, bone marrow, colon, kidneys, bladder, male genitalia

Q: What types of benign pathology will accumulate OncoScint CR/OV?

A: colostomy sites, degenerative joint disease, abdominal aneurysms, postoperative bowel adhesions, local inflammatory lesions

Q: How does delayed imaging help differentiate malignancy from physiologic uptake of OncoScint?

A: tumor becomes more intense with time, physiologic localization washes out

Q: How do hepatic metastases appear on OncoScint CR/OV imaging?

A: cold defects

Q: What agent is available for imaging tumors having somatostatin receptors?

A: ^{111}In-octreotide

Q: What types of tumors can ^{111}I-octreotide image?

A: most neuroendocrine tumors, meningioma, astrocytoma, breast cancer, small cell lung cancer, lymphoma

Q: What is the basic mechanism of uptake of ^{18}F-FDG by malignant tumors?

A: malignant tumors have a higher rate of glycolysis than normal tissue

Q: How is ^{18}F-FDG handled metabolically by cells?

A: it is transported into cells, phosphorylated to ^{18}F-FDG-6-phosphate, which cannot leave the cell, and can undergo no further metabolic degradation

Q: How is ^{18}F-FDG PET imaging useful for the management of astrocytomas?

A: uptake predicts histologic grade, and the scan can be used to detect recurrence and differentiate radiation necrosis from tumor recurrence

Q: How is ^{18}F-FDG PET imaging useful for the management of head/neck tumors?

A: it is more accurate than CT or MRI for detecting the primary tumor and predicting histologic grade

Q: How is ^{18}F-FDG PET imaging useful for the management of breast cancer?

A: it can predict whether primary lesions are benign or malignant and can detect involved axillary lymph nodes

Q: What tracers are used for lymphoscintigraphy?

A: ^{99m}Tc-sulfur colloid (filtered), ^{99m}Tc-human serum albumin (HAS), ^{99m}Tc-antimony colloid, and ^{99m}Tc-dextran

Q: What is a "sentinel node"?

A: The first draining lymph node from a primary cancer

Q: How is lymphoscintigraphy useful in the management of malignant melanoma?

A: lymphoscintigraphy can demonstrate the lymphatic drainage of a primary and the sentinel node and thereby determine which nodes should be resected surgically

Q: Where is the tracer injected for lymphoscintigraphic evaluation of malignant melanoma?

A: intradermally at multiple sites around the skin lesion

Q: How is lymphoscintigraphy useful in the management of breast cancer?

A: lymphoscintigraphy can detect metastatic involvement of the internal mammary lymph nodes

Q: Where is the tracer injected for lymphoscintigraphic evaluation of breast cancer?

A: into the subxiphoid rectus sheath ipsilateral to the midline

Q: How is lymphoscintigraphy useful in the management of prostate carcinoma?

A: lymposcintigraphy can detect metastatic involvement of the internal, common iliac, and para-aortic lymph nodes

Q: Where is the tracer injected for lymphoscintigraphic evaluation of genitourinary tumors?

A: into the ischiorectal fossa

Q: "Your 16-year-old son has just gotten his driver's license. He has never driven the family car without his mother or father beside him. But now, the law says he can, so your son asks for the keys. As he disappears over the horizon, the feeling you get in the pit of your stomach is called . . ."

A: a) *Indygestion*
  b) *Driverticulitis*
  c) *Youth-in-Nausea*
  d) *Dad Nauseam*
  e) *Dyspopseeya*
  f) *Mr. Gutwrench*

Q: ^{67}Ga decays to which element?

A: ^{67}Zn (stable)

Q: Because gallium is excreted in milk, it is recommended to stop breast feeding the infant for _____ .

A: 2 weeks

Q: The biologic half-life of ^{67}Ga citrate is less, more, or equal to the physical half-life?

A: more, 2–3 weeks

Q: The half-time of blood clearance of ^{67}Ga citrate is _____ .

A: less than 3 hr

Q: What fraction of injected ^{67}Ga citrate is excreted from the body after 4 weeks (physical decay is not considered)?

A: one-third

Q: What fraction of ^{67}Ga citrate is absorbed when administered orally?

A: less than 3%

Q: The percentage of injected ^{67}Ga citrate excreted in urine, up to 1 week, is less or more than that excreted in stools?

A: more

Q: The critical organ in ^{67}Ga citrate imaging is _____ .

A: colon

Q: ^{67}Ga negligibly binds to
a. transferrin
b. alpha globulin
c. albumin
d. lactoferrin

A: c

Q: Gallium acts as a physiological analogue of ferric ion. Gallium binds to all of these cells except:
a. lymphocyte
b. neutrophil
c. RBC
d. bacteria

A: c

Q: Gallium does not localize in most adenocarcinomas, except in

_____ .

A: lung and hepatoma

Q: The three clearly established uses of Gallium tumor imaging are

A: metastatic melanoma, hepatoma versus pseudotumor of liver, and monitoring response of lymphoma to chemotherapy

Q: Gallium is taken up by growing tumors or necrotic tumors?

A: growing tumors

Q: Irradiation of tumor may decrease/increase the gallium uptake.

A: decrease

Q: Irradiation of head and neck tumors results in increase/decrease of radiogallium uptake in salivary glands.

A: increase

Q: True/false: Gallium uptake at intramuscular injection site is usually pathological

A: false

Q: True/false: Normal small bowel does not secrete radiogallium.

A: false

Q: Large bowel is one of the normal excretory pathways for radiogallium. The three methods of reducing diagnostic confusion in abdominal imaging are

_____ .

A: gentle cathartics or enema, high-fiber diet, imaging at various intervals

Q: True/false: Gallium is actively bound to siderophores.

A: true

Q: The source of lactoferrin and siderophores, respectively, are
a. lymphocytes
b. leukocytes
c. bacteria
d. fungus
e. tissue macrophage

A: b and c

Q: Lactoferrin is physiologically produced by certain organs that localise gallium. These are
a. lacrimal glands
b. salivary glands
c. breast
d. lactating breast
e. bone
f. liver

A: a, b, c, and d

Q: True/false: Desferoxamine, an iron-chelating agent, is a siderophore.

A: true

Q: Gallium is a physiologic analogue of iron, and it shares iron transport mechanism. However, the main difference between iron and gallium, intracellularly, is _____ .

A: intracellularly bound iron is reduced and incorporated into the cytochrome oxidase transport system, whereas the gallium is trapped intracellularly but not reduced

Q: The gallium-binding affinity of lactoferrin is less/more than that of transferrin.

A: more

Q: For the accuracy of detection of active osteomyelitis,
a. MDP is better than ^{67}Ga
b. ^{67}Ga is better than MDP

A: b

Q: Gallium uptake is usually *not* seen in the following liver disorders:
a. adenoma
b. hemangioma
c. cirrhosis
d. polycystic disease
e. metastasis
f. hepatoma
g. amoebic liver abscess

A: b, c, and d

Q: Lesion detectability by radiogallium is maximum when the lesion size is
a. less than 1 cm
b. 2–5 cm
c. more than 5 cm

A: b

Q: True/false: The accuracy of gallium scan in the evaluation of abdominal disorders is higher in children than in adults.

A: true

Q: The reported highest sensitivity (approximately 100%) of gallium imaging is for _____ .

A: Burkitt's lymphoma, pyogenic acute osteomyelitis (untreated), pyogenic acute arthritis (untreated)

Q: True/false: Discordance of ^{99m}Tc-sulfur colloid and gallium liver images is essential for the diagnosis of hepatoma.

A: true

Q: Positive/negative gallium scan implies poor prognosis in multiple myeloma and neuroblastoma.

A: positive

Q: The gallium scan is positive/negative in acute rheumatoid arthritis

A: positive

Q: Differential diagnosis of negative chest X ray and positive gallium scan include _____ .

A: PCP, cytomegalovirus infection, pulmonary drug toxicity, sarcoidosis, lymphocytic interstitial pneumonitis

Q: Abnormal chest X ray and normal gallium scan of lungs may be seen in _____ . lymphoma

A: Kaposi's sarcoma, pulmonary fibrosis, treated sarcoidosis and inactive tuberculosis

Q: Positive gallium scan and negative computed tomography/ultrasound (CT/US) of abdomen may be seen in _____ .

A: acute inflammation (e.g., peritonitis, pyelonephritis, cystitis)

Match the following six statements with the appropriate antibody structures:
a. antibody fragment
b. whole antibody
c. both
d. neither

Q: major route of clearance is liver

A: b

Q: major route of clearance is kidneys

A: a

Q: most often labeled with ^{111}In chloride

A: b

Q: oncoscint

A: b

Q: may be used to study sites of spread of colorectal carcinoma

A: c

Q: delayed views at several days are feasible

A: b

Q: The most frequent site for recurrence of colorectal carcinoma is:
a. the liver
b. the lungs
c. the extrahepatic abdomen and pelvis
d. the brain

A: c

Q: What percentage of ovarian neoplasms express the TAG-72 antigen?
a. 50%
b. 70%
c. 80%
d. over 90%

A: d

Q: Which of the following is *not* an indication for OncoScint imaging in patients with recurrent colorectal carcinoma?

a. presumed resectable recurrence with no other demonstrable disease
b. routine 1-year follow-up with normal (CEA) and negative work up
c. equivocal findings on CT or MRI
d. unexplained rise of serum CEA with a negative work up

A: b

Q: The MAb B72.3 seeks out what specific antigen in adenocarcinomas?

a. CEA
b. TAG-72
c. both a and b

A: b

Q: "Once upon a time, a Social Security number was all you needed—and all you had. But in 1998, you have a PIN number (or maybe three), a telephone credit card number, a frequent flier number, voice mail access code number, and (hopefully), an E-mail address—all of which you have to memorize, if you know what's good for you. This proliferation of multi-digit numbers in modern life is called . . ."

A: a) *PINitence*
  b) *Code-Dependency*
  c) *Mnemonic Plague*
  d) *Numeralgia*
  e) *Add In-PIN-item*
  f) *Indigitestion*

Q: The FDA-approved and recommended dose of ^{89}Sr for palliating painful bone metastases is:

a. 1–2 mCi
b. 4 mCi
c. 7 mCi
d. 10 mCi

A: b

Q: Following treatment with ^{89}Sr, patients should be in isolation for:

a. 24 hr
b. 48–72 hr
c. at least 5 days
d. isolation not necessary

A: d

Q: True/false: Positive localization on ^{99m}Tc-phosphate bone scan is essential before a painful lesion can be effectively treated with ^{89}Sr.

A: true

Q: Of the following, the metastatic bone lesion least likely to respond to ^{89}Sr palliative therapy is:
a. multiple myeloma
b. prostate carcinoma
c. colon carcinoma
d. breast carcinoma

A: a

Q: The usually administered dose of ^{32}P for treating polycythemia vera is:
a. 1 mCi
b. 2–5 mCi
c. 5–10 mCi
d. 10–15 mCi

A: b

Q: True/false: The effectiveness of ^{32}P therapy in treating polycythemia vera is generally attributed to the marrow suppressive effects of its gamma emissions:

A: false

Q: Besides its use in treating polycythemia vera, some form of ^{32}P has been used to treat:
a. painful bone metastases
b. leukemias
c. malignant pleural effusions
d. all of the above
e. none of the above

A: d

Q: In abscess detection, a false-negative gallium scan may be caused by:
a. patient receiving transfusion
b. polycythemia vera
c. leukopenia
d. a and c
e. all of the above

A: d

Q: True/false: Effective gallium scans can be performed with a low-energy collimator if one utilizes only the 90 and 180 keV gamma photons.

A: false

Match each of the following five statements
with the best choice:
a. ^{67}Ga citrate
b. ^{111}In WBCs
c. both
d. neither

Q: preferable for the study of infectious
disease

A: c

Q: preferable for the detection of
pneumocystis pneumonia in patients
with AIDS

A: a

Q: monchromatic gamma emission

A: d

Q: preferable for study of inflammatory
bowel disease

A: b

Q: effectively detects the presence of
subphrenic abscess

A: c

Q: Studies with both ^{18}F-FDG and ^{11}C
methionine show that metabolites in
malignant lesions are _____
than those in benign lesions.

A: higher

Q: True/false: Increased ^{18}FDG uptake is
found in malignant neoplasms in the lung
of adeno but not in squamous cell types.

A: false

Q: True/false: The lack of increased
uptake of ^{18}FDG in a pulmonary nodule is
a reliable predictor of benignity.

A: true

Q: True/false: PET scanning of the chest
cannot help distinguish between benign
and malignant causes of adenopathy.

A: false

Q: True/false: The lack of morphologic
change of a malignant lesion on CT reliably
predicts a poor response to therapy.

A: false

Q: True/false: Benign breast lesions
accumulate ^{18}FDG to a degree similar to
the surrounding normal breast tissue.

A: true

Q: True/false: One of the medicare
reimbursements approved for PET studies
is to distinguish post-therapy necrosis and
fibrosis from recurrent brain tumor.

A: true

Q: Of the following group of AIDS complications, good gallium uptake is least likely to occur in:
a. mycobacterium infection
b. Hodgkin's disease
c. tuberculous adenopathy
d. Kaposi's sarcoma

A: d

Q: Amyloidosis is most likely to show:
a. positive gallium and positive phosphate uptake
b. positive gallium and negative phosphate uptake
c. negative gallium and positive phosphate uptake
d. negative gallium and negative phosphate uptake

A: c

Q: Normal gallium scan findings at 72 hr may include uptake in all of the following except:
a. salivary glands
b. lacrimal glands
c. liver
d. kidney
e. actually occurs in all of the above

A: d

11 Pulmonary

Q: What is the main indication for ventilation perfusion scintigraphy?

A: evaluation for pulmonary embolism

Q: What is the mortality rate from untreated pulmonary embolism?

A: 30%

Q: Name the two classes of radiopharmaceuticals used for ventilation scintigraphy.

A: radioactive gases and radioaerosols

Q: What three radioactive gases are available for ventilation scintigraphy?

A: ^{127}Xe, ^{133}Xe, ^{81m}Kr

Q: Why can ^{127}Xe be used for postperfusion ventilation scanning?

A: its photon energies are higher than ^{99m}Tc

Q: What is the practical life of an ^{81}Rb-^{81m}Kr generator?

A: about 12 hrs

Q: What is the reason that ^{81m}Kr is not more widely used for ventilation scanning?

A: high costs and impracticality of daily generator replacement

Q: Why can ^{81m}Kr be used for postperfusion imaging?

A: the energy of the principal photon (191 keV) is higher than ^{99m}Tc

Q: Why does xenon accumulate in the livers of some patients?

A: xenon is fat soluble and may accumulate in fatty livers

Q: What is the radiopharmaceutical most commonly used for radioaerosol imaging?

A: ^{99m}Tc-DTPA

Q: What is the appropriate aerosol particle size for radioaerosol ventilation scanning?

A: 1–0.5 microns

Q: What happens to inhaled particles whose size is less than 0.1 microns?

A: they are exhaled and not deposited in the lungs

Q: What happens to inhaled particles whose size is more than 2–3 microns?

A: they settle in the large airways

Q: How can both ventilation and perfusion imaging be performed with the same isotope?

A: the dose of the second study must be substantially greater than the first

Q: What is the usual adult dosage for a ventilation scan with xenon?

A: 10–20 mCi

Q: What are the three phases of a xenon ventilation study?

A: wash-in (first breath), equilibrium, wash-out

Q: What view is most commonly taken for a xenon ventilation study?

A: posterior chest

Q: What does the patient breathe during the wash-in portion of a xenon-ventilation study?

A: radioactive xenon mixed with air

Q: What does the patient breathe during the equilibrium portion of a xenon-ventilation study?

A: radioactive xenon mixed with air

Q: What does the patient breathe during the washout portion of a xenon-ventilation study?

A: air without radioactive xenon

Q: How much of the activity in a nebulizer is delivered to the lungs in a radioaerosol ventilation study?

A: 5–10%

Q: How much radioactivity is typically placed in the nebulizer for a radioaerosol ventilation study?

A: 25–27 mCi

Q: What is the biologic half-life of inhaled ^{99m}Tc-DTPA in the lung?

A: about 1 hr

Q: How does ^{99m}Tc-MAA localize in the lung?

A: after intravenous injection, ^{99m}Tc-MAA is trapped in the pulmonary vascular bed on the first pass

Q: Why does ^{99m}Tc-MAA uptake in the lung reflect lung blood flow?

A: areas of reduced perfusion have less tracer delivered during the first-pass injection

Q: What is the biologic half-life of ^{99m}Tc-MAA in the lung?

A: 2–3 hr

Q: What is the differential diagnosis of systemic organ uptake of ^{99m}Tc-MAA?

A: free pertechnetate or a right-to-left shunt

Q: What is the best organ to image to detect right-to-left shunting of ^{99m}Tc-MAA?

A: the brain

Q: What is the problem with administering too few particles of ^{99m}Tc-MAA?

A: the pattern of uptake is not based on a statistically valid distribution of particles to reflect blood flow

Q: What is the problem with administering too many particles of ^{99m}Tc-MAA?

A: it may cause hemodynamic obstruction

Q: What is the minimum number of particles of ^{99m}Tc-MAA that should be injected for a perfusion scan?

A: 60,000

Q: What group of patients should always get the minimum number of particles of ^{99m}Tc-MAA?

A: patients with pulmonary hypertension

Q: How do you adjust the number of particles of ^{99m}Tc-MAA that are administered to a patient?

A: adjust the activity of ^{99m}Tc-pertechnetate

Q: How will the number of particles of ^{99m}Tc-MAA that are administered to a patient change with decay of the kit?

A: the number of particles required to give a dose increases with decay

Q: What is the usual dose of ^{99m}Tc-MAA for a lung perfusion scan?

A: 2–5 mCi

Q: How long after injection of ^{99m}Tc-MAA can imaging for a lung perfusion scan begin?

A: immediately

Q: What is the minimum number of counts that should be obtained for a lung perfusion scan?

A: 500,000

Q: What may occur if blood clots form in the syringe used to inject ^{99m}Tc-MAA for a lung perfusion scan?

A: hot spots may appear in the lung

Q: What should you do with a syringe containing ^{99m}Tc-MAA just before injecting it into a patient?

A: the syringe should be agitated to prevent sedimentation of the particles; if the particles sediment, they may be left in the syringe after injection

Q: What is the normal pattern of uptake on the wash-in and equilibrium phases of a ^{133}Xe lung ventilation scan?

A: homogenous uptake throughout both lungs

Q: What is the normal half-time of washout of ^{133}Xe from the lungs during the washout phase of a lung ventilation scan?

A: 2 min or less

Q: What can cause diffusely delayed washout of ^{133}Xe from the lungs during the washout phase of a lung ventilation scan in a normal patient?

A: difficulty breathing through the apparatus for delivering xenon

Q: What two organs outside the chest can show uptake of ^{133}Xe in a lung ventilation scan performed on a normal person?

A: the stomach (due to swallowed gas) and the liver; if uptake in the liver is prominent, a fatty liver should be suspected

Q: What two organs outside the chest can show uptake of ^{99m}Tc-DTPA in a lung ventilation scan performed on a normal person?

A: the stomach (due to swallowed aerosol) and the kidneys

Q: What parts of the lung may be seen on an aerosol scan, but will never be seen on a lung ventilation scan performed c̄ gas?

A: the trachea and large airways

Q: What are two photopenic areas that will be seen in lung perfusion scans of normal patients?

A: the heart and the lung hila

Q: What is a ventilation perfusion mismatch?

A: the perfusion defect does not correspond to a ventilation scan abnormality

Q: What is the difference between a segmental and a nonsegmental perfusion defect on a perfusion Q scan?

A: a segmental defect reflects the vascular territory of a pulmonary artery branch; nonsegmental defects do not

Q: What is the name for the most commonly used criteria for diagnosing pulmonary emboli on a V/Q scan?

A: PIOPED criteria

Q: What are the four diagnostic categories for pulmonary embolism with a V/Q scan?

A: normal, low probability, intermediate probability, and high probability

Q: What is the typical appearance of a low-probability V/Q scan?

A: matched ventilation perfusion abnormalities without corresponding radiographic findings

Q: In the PIOPED trial the probability of pulmonary embolism in a patient with a low probability V/Q scan ranges from _____ .

A: 5–20%

Q: What is the probability of pulmonary embolism in a patient with normal lung perfusion?

A: less than 1%

Q: What is the probability of pulmonary embolism in a patients with a high-probability V/Q scan and a high clinical suspicion of pulmonary embolism?

A: 96%

Q: What is the likelihood of a patient with a normal- or low-probability V/Q scan who does not get anticoagulated of having an adverse event due to an untreated pulmonary embolism?

A: <1%; in the PIOPED study, no such complications were detected

Q: What is the most common cause of a false-positive V/Q scan for acute pulmonary embolism?

A: unresolved chronic pulmonary embolism

Q: What factors predispose to rapid and complete resolution of pulmonary emboli?

A: young age, small emboli, no comorbid conditions

Q: How fast can pulmonary emboli resolve?

A: 1 day

Q: How long can it take for pulmonary emboli to resolve?

A: they can last for the life of the patient

Q: How can the pattern of a perfusion scan in a patient with pulmonary embolism change without new emboli?

A: proximal clots can break up and lodge more peripherally

Q: What is a stripe sign on a V/Q scan, and what is its meaning?

A: preservation of blood flow at the pleural margin of a perfusion defect; pulmonary emboli usually cause perfusion abnormalities that extend to the pleural margin and imply a low probability for pulmonary embolism

Q: What is the appearance of a large amount of pleural fluid on a V/Q scan on a supine patient?

A: the pleural fluid uniformly attenuates the lung in the posterior images, but not in the anterior images

Q: What is the fissure sign on a V/Q scan?

A: a perfusion defect along a pleural fissure due to pleural fluid in the fissure

Q: How can a perfusion scan be used to manage patients with lung cancer who are candidates for surgical resection?

A: quantitation of the scan can be used to predict postoperative pulmonary function based on the extent of surgery

Q: How can deep venous thrombosis be detected with radionuclide venography?

A: the patient's feet can be injected with ^{99m}Tc-MAA and obstruction of the thigh veins detected

Q: "You're posing for a photograph. Even though you've been warned 1,000 times, you still can't resist looking at the flash as it goes off. The resulting visual butterflies is called . . ."

A: a) *Lumen-aeries*
   b) *Lepidopticals*
   c) *Shutterflies*
   d) *Flashtroentereyetis*
   e) *Cornea-opias*

Q: The most commonly used radiotracer for perfusion imaging is _____ , whose particle size must be greater than _____ microns but less than _____ microns.

A: ^{99m}Tc-MAA, 8, 100

Q: An alternative perfusion agent is _____ , which has the advantage of a _____ , but the disadvantage of _____ .

A: ^{99m}Tc-HAM (human albumin, microspheres, more uniform particle size, a higher incidence of allergic reactions

Q: For perfusion studies, tracer is injected intravenously with the patient in the _____ position and imaged in _____ position.

A: supine, any

Q: Why should ^{99m}Tc-MAA for a lung perfusion scan be injected with the patient supine?

A: if the patient is upright, there may be a basilar predominance of perfusion

Q: Why is position during injection important?

A: to more evenly distribute the pulmonary blood flow

Q: True/false: Normal pulmonary perfusion is relatively greater in the lung bases. Why?

A: true; because of the gravity

Q: The average range of microspheres is _____ , of MAA, _____ .

A: 20–40 microns, 10–100 microns

Q: Approximately _____ of the pulmonary capillary bed is occluded during a lung scan.

A: 1/1000

Q: State the physical half-life and photon energy of ^{133}Xe.

A: 5 days, 80keV

Q: State the photon energy of ^{81m}Kr.

A: 190 keV

Q: List four advantages of ^{133}Xe.

A: inexpensive, readily available, good shelf life, includes washout phase that increases sensitivity for obstructive airway disease

Q: List five disadvantages of ^{133}Xe:

A: poor image quality, high absorbed radiation dose, difficult to obtain multiple views, difficult to perform in uncooperative patients, requires shielding

Q: List five advantages of ^{81m}Kr:

A: high photon energy, multiple views, low pt rad dose, can obtain ventilation after perfusion study, simultaneous acquisition perfusion and ventilation, easy to perform even in ventilator assisted patients

Q: Name three disadvantages of ^{81m}Kr:

A: limited availability, expensive, no washout phase

Q: List five advantages of radioaerosols (^{99m}Tc-DTPA):

A: inexpensive, readily available, multiple views, possible to obtain ventilation after perfusion study, administration of tracer can be performed in ventilator-assisted patients

Q: List three disadvantages of aerosols:

A: no washout phase, may obtain poor images due to central deposition, does not permit simultaneous (V/Q) image acquisition

Q: ^{81m}Kr with a half-life of _____ is the product of _____ , which has a physical half-life of _____ .

A: 13 sec, 81 Rb, 4.7 hr

Q: True/false: ^{81m}Kr is generator produced.

A: true

Q: True/false: ^{81}Rb is cyclotron produced.

A: true

Q: True/false: Albumin macroaggregates remain in the pulmonary capillary bed for weeks, limiting the number of follow-up perfusion scans that can be safely performed.

A: false

Q: The particles used for perfusion imaging are removed from the lung by _____ .

A: phagocytosis

Q: True/false: The biologic half-life of MAA is longer than that of albumin microspheres.

A: false

Q: Using ^{133}Xe as the ventilation agent, ventilation precedes perfusion. Why?

A: Tc has a higher gamma energy, resulting in down-scatter degrading the Xe image

Q: What is the advantage of acquiring both ventilation and perfusion simultaneously?

A: ensures corresponding positions for ventilation and perfusion

Q: Is a dual-headed camera necessary for simultaneous V/Q imaging?

A: no; dual peak with one head is adequate

Q: True/false: In a patient with a *high* pretest probability of pulmonary embolism (PE), the negative predictive value of a normal scan exceeds 95%.

A: true

Q: True/false: In a patient with a *low* pretest probability of PE, the positive predictive value of a positive scan exceeds 95%.

A: false

Q: Signs and symptoms of PE included in the "classic" triad are _____ , _____ , and _____ .

A: dyspnea, pleuritic chest pain, hemoptysis

Q: True/false: The presence of this triad has a positive predictive value for pulmonary embolism exceeding 95%.

A: false

Q: True/false: V/Q scanning is nondiagnostic in most patients with pulmonary edema.

A: false

Q: True/false: Most patients with PE show infiltrate or effusion on properly exposed chest X rays.

A: false

Q: According to the PIOPED interpretive criteria, a small perfusion defect comprises less than _____ of a lung segment.

A: 25%

Q: A large perfusion defect comprises at least _____ of a lung segment.

A: 75%

Q: Patients with normal chest X rays with small perfusion defects (even with vent mismatch) on lung scans have _____ probability scans for PE.

A: low

Q: Patients with normal chest X rays with (V/P) matched defects have a _____ probability scan for PE.

A: low

Q: A patient with a segmental perfusion defect substantially smaller than a corresponding radiographic abnormality (V irrelevant) have a _____ probability scan for PE.

A: low

Q: A segmental perfusion defect the same size as a chest X ray and vent abnormality ("triple match") represents an _____ probability scan for PE.

A: indeterminate

Q: A single moderate-sized perfusion defect (nl chest X ray and vent) represents an _____ probability scan for PE.

A: intermediate

Q: Other cases of V/P mismatch include (other than acute PE) _____ .

A: old PE, nonthrombotic emboli, vasculitis, prior (RT), bronchogenic (CA), inactive (TB), (AV) malformation, lymphoma, fibrosa mediastinitis, sarcoidosis, pulmonary hypertension, vascular compression by enlarged hilar nodes

Q: True/false: Absence of perfusion to an entire lung is common with PE.

A: false

Q: Absence of perfusion to an entire lung should suggest _____ .

A: central vascular compression by tumor

Q: A pneumectomy patient may develop respiratory insufficiency if the post-op forced expiratory volume in 1 sec (Fev 1) is less than_____ .

A: 0.8 liters

Q: Split function studies determine the counts in each lung in anterior and posterior views by computing the _____ .

A: arithmetic mean counts

Q: The post-op Fev 1.0 is predicted by multiplying the _____ by the fraction of the counts contributed by the lung that will not be removed.

A: pre-op Fev 1.0

Q: In lung scanning, the "stripe sign" generally is reflective of:
a. pulmonary emboli
b. nonembolic disease such as chronic obstructive pulmonary disease
c. pulmonary venous hypertension
d. pleural fluid

A: b

Q: Matched absence or near absence of perfusion and ventilation in an entire lung may be associated with:
a. lung carcinoma
b. aspirated foreign body
c. Swyer-James syndrome
d. all of the above
e. none of the above

A: d

Q: A reversal of pulmonary blood flow with the upper lobes receiving more perfusion than the lower lobes is most often associated with:
a. interstitial fibrosis
b. pulmonary emboli
c. pleural fluid
d. pulmonary venous hypertension

A: d

Q: The percentage of pulmonary emboli that proceed to infarction is approximately:
a. 0–5%
b. 5–15%
c. 20–30%
d. 30–40%
e. >40%

A: b

Match the five following findings with the scintigraphic interpretation:
a. low probability lung scan
b. intermediate lung scan
c. high probability lung scan

Q: clear chest X ray and multiple matched V/Q defects

A: a

Q: single segmental V/Q mismatch

A: b

Q: perfusion defect <radiographic infiltrate

A: a

Q: multiple subsegmental defects

A: a

Q: lobar V/Q mismatch

A: c

Q: perfusion defect equal to radiographic infiltrate

A: b

Match the five following statements with the appropriate ventilation lung agent:

a. ^{81m}Kr
b. ^{99m}Tc-DTPA particles
c. ^{133}Xe

Q: associated with the lowest radiation dose   **A:** a

Q: 5-day physical half-life   **A:** c

Q: study generally is performed only in one position   **A:** c

Q: may be effectively performed following the perfusion study   **A:** a

Q: often causes central "hot spots" in emphysematous patients   **A:** b

Q: The visualization of the kidneys on a ^{99m}Tc-MAA perfusion lung scan can be caused by: **A:** e

a. right-to-left shunting
b. free ^{99m}Tc
c. MAA particles less than 10 microns in size
d. a and c
e. all of the above